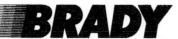

TAIGMAN'S
ADVANCED CARDIOLOGY
(In Plain English)

Syd Canan

Charly D. Miller

Mike Taigman

BRADY
Prentice Hall
Upper Saddle River, New Jersey 07458

Production Editor: *Cathy O'Connell*
Interior Design and Layout: *Lightworks Design*
Cover Design: *Mary Jo DeFranco*
Prepress/Manufacturing Buyer: *Ilene Sanford*
Acquisitions Editor: *Susan Katz*
Editorial Assistant: *Carol Sobel*

NOTICE ON CARE PROCEDURES

It is the intent of the authors and publisher that this textbook be used as part of a formal education program taught by qualified instructors and supervised by a licensed physician. The procedures described in this textbook are based upon consultation with EMT and medical authorities. The authors and publisher have taken care to make certain that these procedures reflect currently accepted clinical practice; however, they cannot be considered absolute recommendations.

The material in this textbook contains the most current information available at the time of publication. However, federal, state, and local guidelines concerning clinical practices, including without limitation, those governing infection control and universal precautions, change rapidly. The reader should note, therefore, that the new regulations may require changes in some procedures.

It is the responsibility of the reader to familiarize himself or herself with the policies and procedures set by federal, state and local agencies as well as the institution or agency where the reader is employed. The authors and the publisher of this textbook and the supplements written to accompany it disclaim any liability, loss or risk resulting directly or indirectly from the suggested procedures and theory, from any undetected errors, or from the reader's misunderstanding of the text. It is the reader's responsibility to stay informed of any new changes or recommendations made by any federal, state, and local agency as well as by his or her employing institution or agency.

Printed in the United States of America

ISBN 0-89303-999-3

Prentice-Hall International (UK) Limited,London
Prentice-Hall of Australia Pty. Limited, Sydney
Prentice-Hall Canada Inc., Toronto
Prentice-Hall Hispanoamericana, S.A., Mexico
Prentice-Hall of India Private Limited, New Delhi
Prentice-Hall of Japan, Inc., Tokyo
Pearson Education Asia Pte. Ltd., Singapore
Editora Prentice-Hall do Brasil, Ltda., Rio de Janeiro

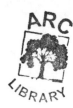

This book is due on the last date stamped below.
Failure to return books on the date due may result
in assessment of overdue fees.

	FINES	.50 per day	

Contents

Preface

When I was educated as a paramedic, there was a message that my classmates and I heard loudly, clearly, and often from our instructors. Whenever we'd ask questions about things that weren't covered in our class objectives, we were told, "Paramedics don't need to know that." And when it came to EKGs, we were told that a lot. Everytime we asked about bundle branch blocks, or axis, or myocardial infarction, and the like, we were told, "Paramedics don't need to know that." But as soon as we started taking care of patients, we discovered that our patients hadn't read our paramedic textbooks. Our patients didn't limit their emergencies to the objectives we had been taught. In fact, they often presented with complaints or signs and symptoms that seemed to be related to things paramedics "don't need to know."

Along that same line of thought, it's a misnomer to call this text "Advanced EKGs." In the world of sick people there are people who can read EKGs (and base therapeutic decisions upon them) and people who cannot. So, in 1981, a group of us got together and developed a workshop designed to help paramedics learn all the things about EKGs that they actually did need to know but hadn't been previously taught—things that were necessary for them to provide safe and comprehensive care to their patients.

Over the years the workshop audience changed and grew in an interesting manner. As paramedics began exhibiting "advanced" abilities to interpret and respond to EKGs, critical care nurses took notice. Many of them discovered the workshop to be a surprisingly clear way to finally understand things that were previously taught to them in a complex and confusing manner. Soon, emergency department and medical control physicians began attending the workshop in order to better understand the radio reports of the paramedics who were bringing them well-treated patients!

In 1988, we presented one of our three-day Advanced Cardiology workshops in Broomfield, Colorado. On the first day, seated in the front row, was a very energetic participant whom I later learned was named Charly Miller. She asked if it would be okay if she tape-recorded the workshop. Of course we gave her permission to do so, and then we didn't think much more about it.

A few months later, Charly came to the Denver General Paramedic Division, where I was employed, to do a "ride-along." When she showed up for her shift, she handed me a thick manila envelope that contained a word-for-word transcription of the three 8-hour days of the Broomfield EKG workshop. She said, "I don't know—maybe you can use this for something someday."

A little bit of time passed. I left regular street work and moved to Florida to take an EMS management job. At that same time, Charly was hired as a Denver General Paramedic. She also began her writing career then and had published several EMS-oriented textbooks before we ran across each other again at an EMS conference in Colorado Springs, Colorado.

It was there that Charly asked me, "Do you ever think of turning your EKG workshop into a textbook? The industry really needs it, you know."

And I said, "Yeah. But it would be a lot of work."

To which she replied, "Well, I'm gonna write your book, do you want to be part of it?"

How could I refuse?

Then, knowing that we would need some creative (and reality based) direction, we immediately involved my good friend and long time co-author, Syd Canan, in the project. And that's how this text was launched.

This is actually not a "textbook," but a "workshop on paper." As such, we have worked hard to preserve the spirit and spontaneity that accompanies a live interaction. This text is not intended to give an exhaustive view of everything to do with cardiology. Rather, it is intended to provide a solid, useful, real-world understanding of the emergency electrocardiogram and its relationship to sick patients. It focuses most heavily on EKG-influenced decisions that critically affect whether or not patients survive their medical emergencies and what kind of lifestyle they might have upon discharge.

This workshop-on-paper, like its live counterpart, presumes that its participants will have a basic understanding of electrocardiography. Waveform recognition, ability to do measurements, and basic EKG terminology are background skills that participants (and readers) are presumed to already have.

A few years ago I heard Tom Peters speak at a conference. He is the author of *In Search of Excellence, A Passion for Excellence, Thriving on Chaos,* and *Liberation Management.* There were 6,000 people in the audience, and each had paid $90.00 to hear Tom Peters speak for 2 hours. Mr. Peters' introductory remark was, "I pride myself on never having had an original thought." And, in that spirit, most of what is contained in our electrocardiography workshop, and in this text, is *not* the creation of the authors. It is almost entirely based on the research, writings, and teachings of two well-respected cardiologists.

The first of these is Dr. Henry J. L. Marriott. Dr. Marriott is probably the world's foremost author and educator of electrocardiography. He has presented hundreds of advanced EKG workshops for critical care nurses and cardiologists. He has written numerous articles, research papers, and textbooks on the subject. Much of our text consists of adaptations and translations of Dr. Marriott's work that have been geared to the prehospital audience. If it were not for his eloquent ability to communicate and his generosity with information, our workshop (and text) would never have been developed. Unless indicated otherwise, Dr. Marriott's text *Practical Electrocardiography,* 8th Edition (Williams & Wilkins, Baltimore, 1988) provides the reference for our presented material.

Our other mentor, educator, and facilitator for this text is Dr. Gerald Gordon. When paramedic programs first started in Colorado, Dr. Gordon decided that he wanted paramedics to be able to handle *anything.* In fact, his first paramedic courses were almost two years long! In them, he covered cardiology in such depth that graduates of his program were regularly consulted by emergency room and internal medicine physicians for their emergency room electrocardiogram interpretive abilities (whether or not the graduates had delivered the patients in question). Dr. Gordon's adherence to detail and focus on the well-being of the patient have greatly influenced this text.

As you read and experience this text, keep in mind that "all things change." We have done our best to provide up-to-date and plain English explanations of the electrocardiogram and its impact on patient treatment. However, the world of medicine (and electrocardiography in particular) is one of ever-altering thoughts and theories. It is the responsibility of every "advanced" care provider to keep abreast of new discoveries and developments concerning patient care protocols. We anticipate that this text will allow providers to feel more comfortable with their understanding of electrocardiography and how (and why) care changes develop.

Mike Taigman

TERMINOLOGY NOTE

Although, it is traditional for texts to be prefaced with statements regarding the use of "he" versus "she," in this text we instead need to discuss the use of "ECG" versus "EKG" and "arrhythmia" versus "dysrhythmia."

Certainly, ECG is the literal abbreviation for electrocardiogram. And the term EKG was introduced—at least according to my recollection of medical folklore—to deal with the problem of illegible handwriting on the part of many physicians. Apparently, what often happened was that a physician would order an electrocardiogram (ECG) for a patient. But, because of poor handwriting, the order was misinterpreted as EEG. Not surprisingly, it was difficult to make cardiotherapeutic decisions based on a tracing of a patient's brain waves. Consequently, the term EKG was adopted to more clearly differentiate between the two and has since become traditional and commonplace. (It also reflects the abbreviation for the German version of the word: elektrokardiogram.) The move to return to ECG reeks of medical snobbery, and we refuse to submit!* Thus, the term EKG will be used throughout this text.

Similar upstarts have suggested that the term "dysrhythmia" is much more proper than the term "arrhythmia." We suspect that those who relentlessly pursue this quibbling debate over linguistic definitions are people who know which direction toilet paper is supposed to unfold from the rolls, people who clean their plates at the end of every meal, and people who have matching socks neatly laid out in color-coordinated rows in their dresser drawer. These people are not us. We are paramedics. Consequently, throughout this text we will be using the more common and easier to utter term arrhythmia, rather than dysrhythmia.

Finally, all patient names used in this text are totally fictitious. If by any chance a name and medical event resemble those of known persons, living or dead, it is pure coincidence.

---

* After reading our text, Dr. Marriot would like to interject the following: "'ECG' is *not* 'snobbery'—it is simply speaking *English* instead of *Dutch*!"

Acknowledgments

From Mike Taigman: I would like to gratefully acknowledge Charly Miller (for doing most of the "hard" work related to this text) and Syd Canan (for keeping us on track while we translated the spoken word into written word). I would also like to acknowledge the co-instructors who have participated in the cardiology workshop over the years: Tony Head, paramedic; Greg Mullen, paramedic; and Linda Larson, RN. To Kate Dernocoeur, who helps me realize that writing is no more difficult than reading EKGs as long as you have a systematic approach, thank you. To my "brother," Thom Dick, thank you for constantly reminding me that if we don't take good care of ourselves we can't take good care of sick people. And to all those professionals who have participated in our workshops over the years, later using what they learned to provide good care for sick hearts, thank you all!

From Syd Canan: Syd gratefully acknowledges Mike Taigman for some of the heartiest friendship a person could wish for (as well as for helping create a worthy and successful writing partnership). Syd also wishes to acknowledge co-author Charly Miller for having the gumption to tackle this project. Finally, Syd acknowledges family and loved ones—you know who you are!

From Charly D. Miller: Charly extends her heartfelt gratitude to her co-authors: Mike, thank you for at least pretending to flinch when I tried to "crack the whip." But, sincerely, thank-you for providing the EKG material— in English—we've all needed for so long. Syd, I couldn't have done this without you! You'll never know how incredibly important you were to this text. Finally, I'd like to thank David, my personal "ghost" co-author and spousal unit for everything.

SPECIAL CREDIT

Several case studies within this text were previously presented in JEMS (*Journal of Emergency Medical Services*). From approximately 1986 to 1992, Mike and Syd co-authored an occasional JEMS column entitled "Cardiology Practicum," which introduced many of the concepts of advanced cardiology to a national audience. The authors gratefully acknowledge JEMS' contribution to the development of prehospital electrocardiographic skills and their cooperation with this project.

About the Authors

Mike Taigman has been involved in prehospital emergency medicine since 1974. He became fascinated with EKGs early in his career, spending two years studying them on his own before he was old enough to go to paramedic school. In 1981, Mike gathered a small group of instructors together and presented the first Advanced EKG Workshop for prehospital professionals. Since that time, the workshop has grown and adapted and has been presented to medical professionals, including paramedics, critical care nurses, and emergency medical physicians, throughout the United States and Canada. Along with co-author, Syd Canan, Mike has published dozens of advanced EKG articles in JEMS (*Journal of Emergency Medical Services*). They were called "Cardiology Practicum." Mike continues to lecture and write on a variety of EMS-related subjects worldwide.

Syd Canan is a paramedic with nearly 20 years of experience in EMS. EKGs didn't come into Syd's life until 1977 and have never been an easy skill for this shy individual. But, since first learning to decipher those "squiggly little lines," Syd's mission has been to convince others of the importance of reading multiple leads in the field. Syd realized that simple souls can—and should—work everyday to master this stuff. And working with Mike Taigman has always been a great pleasure.

Charly D. Miller is *not* a cardiologist—and is proud of it! She is a field paramedic, currently employed by Denver General Paramedic Division. Ever since being "rescued" from the confusion created by various cardiology texts by Mike Taigman's Advanced EKG Workshop, Charly has been determined to bring this text into being. Now, at last, no paramedic will again be forced to suffer through annoying "cardiologese" to obtain a clear and useful understanding of multiple-lead EKGs.

CHAPTER 1

Atrial-Ventricular Heart Blocks

The description and classification of atrial-ventricular (A-V) heart blocks has often been the source of much controversy and confusion. This book begins with A-V blocks in order to highlight the importance of mastering this challenging topic.

The paradigms surrounding A-V heart blocks must be changed. A paradigm ("pair´-a-dime") is a belief system. When you have a belief system, everything you experience gets filtered through it. For instance, if you have the belief system that people with long hair and beards are hippies and use dope, then every experience that you have with long-haired, bearded people (like myself) will be affected by that belief system. You'd think, "Well, he probably said that because he's been smoking marijuana for too long." In reality, I'm probably one of the "straightest" people in America! I don't even drink.

Traditionally, people have learned that A-V heart blocks are classified as first-degree, second-degree, or third-degree heart blocks. Well, in most areas of medicine, when you think of a disease process in terms of "degrees," you usually think of an increasing severity of disease that directly corresponds to each increasing number. For instance, a patient with third-degree burns is more severely injured than a patient with second-degree burns on the same area of the body. And a patient with second-degree burns is certainly more severely injured than one with the same extent of first-degree burns.

The treatment received by these patients is also directly related to the degree of their burns. A patient with third-degree burns requires more significant treatment than a patient with "only" first-degree burns. And so on.

1

When such labels are applied to A-V heart blocks, the same progressive degree of severity is inferred. *This inference is false.* Many electrocardiograms (EKGs) that are labeled third-degree heart blocks are not life-threatening and reflect less disease process than those showing second-degree heart blocks. And some patients with first-degree heart blocks actually have a significant extent of disease.

Because of the corresponding "degree" of treatment rendered, this mislabeling has often led to mismanagement. Patients with A-V heart blocks have often been either undertreated or overtreated. Unfortunately, this has caused some patients to survive with impaired life-styles or to die when they didn't have to.

To change the belief system surrounding A-V heart blocks, we need to effect a paradigm shift. This shift incorporates the reclassification of A-V blocks that were designed and introduced by Henry Marriott in the early 1980s.[1] This classification consists of a complete set of guidelines that makes it a lot easier to identify and treat A-V heart blocks.

If you know anyone who has tried to lose weight, quit smoking, quit drinking, start an exercise program, or make any other kind of significant change in their life or life-style, you've probably seen the stress that goes along with making a change. For some people, the old-and-familiar is preferable to something new, even if it doesn't work very well. But those who are willing to venture into this new territory of A-V heart block classifications will be rewarded with a clearer understanding of EKGs and a better ability to care for patients with sick hearts.

First, let's be sure that we're clear on the definition of the term *block*. Block is defined as the failure of conduction due to a disease process. Rate or refractory factors that interfere with conduction do not constitute a block.

For example, examine the atrial rate of the EKG strip in Figure 1.1. The atrial rate is approximately 250 beats per minute. What do you think is pathologically wrong with an A-V node that won't let the ventricles beat at the rate of 250 times per minute? If you answered, "nothing," you're absolutely right. This is not a block, this is 2:1 A-V conduction. The word block doesn't belong here.

Here's another one.

Some people have called Figure 1.2 "Atrial flutter with 4:1 A-V block." It shows an unusually fast flutter rate, about 425 beats per minute. Again, there is nothing pathologically wrong with an A-V node that protects its ventricles from having to beat 425 times per minute. The node is actually doing its job. There would be something wrong if the A-V node allowed the ventricles to beat that fast! So, before using the term block, you need to consider both the atrial and ventricular rates. Remember that block is defined as the failure of conduction due to a disease process.

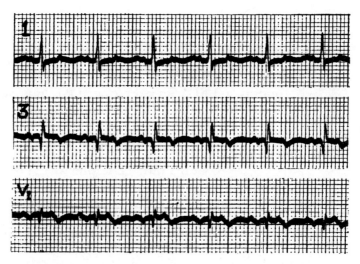

FIGURE 1.1 (Henry J. L. Marriott: *Practical Electrocardiography,* 8th ed., 1988; Williams & Wilkins, Baltimore.)

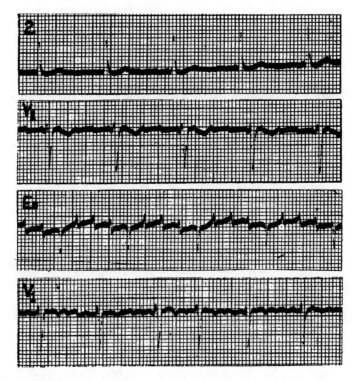

FIGURE 1.2 (Henry J. L. Marriott: *Practical Electrocardiography,* 8th ed., 1988; Williams & Wilkins, Baltimore.)

PROLONGED P-R INTERVAL

The first in the reclassification of A-V heart blocks is the *prolonged P-R interval.* Any EKG with a constant P-R interval of greater than 0.20 seconds is an EKG with a prolonged P-R interval.

Prolonged P-R Interval Rule

Any EKG with a P-R interval of greater than 0.20 seconds.

We previously learned to call this a "first-degree A-V block." We also learned that first-degree A-V block is, for the most part, nothing to worry about. Usually, the presence of a first-degree A-V block does not figure into medication decisions, transportation decisions, or anything else. Why did we learn about it then? To be tested, maybe?

Let's consider a case involving a prolonged P-R interval. An 80-year-old female had a syncopal episode while walking down a flight of stairs. She whacked her head when she hit the bottom. Her husband called 911.

When the paramedic crew got there, her husband told them the story and described a brief loss of consciousness, saying that she had been confused since she "woke up." The paramedics immobilized her spine, gave her oxygen, and started a prophylactic intravenous line. She arrived at the hospital unconscious, responsive only to painful stimuli, with a very slow respiratory rate. Her blood pressure was 140/100.

The paramedics who brought this woman in had run only a lead II strip in the field. Because the base line was too choppy to clearly see any atrial activity, they diagnosed her rhythm as atrial fibrillation. I happened to be in the emergency department doing a clinical rotation for paramedic school. The doctor on duty grabbed me and said, "The paramedic's EKG diagnosis in that room is wrong. Go figure out what the right one is."

Although apprehensive, I eagerly went in and ran leads I, II, III, and MCL_1. The baseline was choppy in all those leads because the woman had fine tremors from posturing due to her head injury. However, I noticed that the QRS complexes were perfectly regular. I asked myself, "What's the hallmark of atrial fibrillation? Irregularly irregular QRS complexes." So I figured that the regular QRS complexes must be the reason that the doctor believed this was not atrial fibrillation. But I needed to be able to see the atrial activity to decide what this really was. Not to be daunted, I remembered to run an S_5 lead.

When you can't see atrial activity on an EKG and you think it might be hidden, run a strip from the S_5 lead. Place one electrode on the manubrium, immediately below the suprasternal notch. Place the other electrode in the fifth intercostal space, just to the right of the sternum. (By convention, the negative lead is at the manubrium, but it actually makes little difference which is positive and which is negative.) This lead placement effectively places the leads on either side of the atria. If there is any

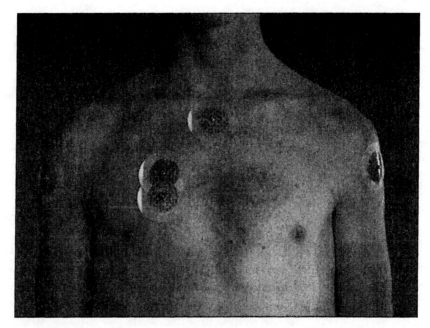

PHOTO 1.1 S₅ lead placement. (Michal Heron, photographer.)

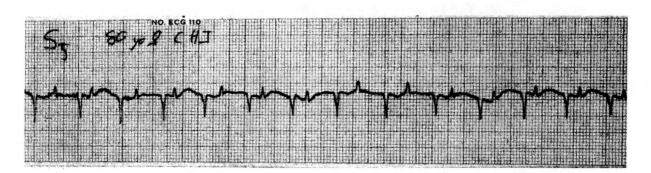

FIGURE 1.3

atrial activity at all, this lead gives you your best chance of obtaining a clear view of it. Figure 1.3 is the strip that I obtained with the S₅ lead placement.

Sometimes, when I show this to people, they say, "well, those are just pointy little T waves!" Now, how do you decide whether something is P waves or T waves? Ah, ha! The Q-T interval.

As Marriott so aptly puts it, determining "who's married to whom" is an important diagnostic determination in cases like this. Every T wave should be a fixed and constant distance from its QRS complex. Is there any reason that a T wave would vary in its distance from the QRS? Not when the rate is constant and regular. So each Q-T interval should be the same.

You can see that the waves in Figure 1.3 vary in distance from the QRS. Look at the Q-T interval after the first QRS. It's about six little boxes long. But the Q-T interval after the second QRS is only about three and a half little boxes long. Thus they can't be T waves.

On the other hand, if you consider those waves to be P waves and measure the distance to the following QRS, you will find a fixed and constant P-R interval. And when you measure it, it's about 0.36 seconds long. That's an unusually long P-R interval.

When you originally learned about "first-degree A-V heart block," were you were taught to be concerned? Probably not. It was probably considered "no big deal." In the case of our elderly woman, the paramedics fortunately had obtained a detailed history of her fall. Her husband said, "We were just walking down the stairs.... She was walking in front of me, and, it's like, she passed out and then fell.... She didn't trip or catch her heel—nothing like that."

The patient had a syncopal episode and fell down the stairs. And she ended up requiring surgery to evacuate a good-sized subdural hematoma. But before she went into the operating room, the emergency department physician considered the history of her fall. Looking at her very prolonged P-R interval, he recognized that a possible reason for her syncopal episode may have been a transient episode of higher-level A-V block and bradycardia. So he put in a pacemaker before she went into surgery. Few physicians would have considered placing a pacemaker in a patient with a "simple" first-degree heart block. This lady was lucky.

The next day, when I came in for another clinical rotation, I visited her in the neurotrauma intensive care unit (ICU). Her monitor displayed a complete heart block that was being paced by the pacemaker inserted the day before. Her chart said that, during this serious neurosurgical procedure, she progressed from a prolonged P-R interval to a complete heart block. Her ventricular rate dropped to 32. When this happened, they simply activated her pacemaker and the surgery continued.

When this 80-year-old woman went into complete heart block with a ventricular rate of 32, how well do you imagine she would have done without the pacemaker? She may not have survived. This is a case of what would previously have been called a "first-degree heart block," which was actually much more ominous than the term implies. It happened to be an indication for a pacemaker. The point is this: every EKG needs to be considered within the context of the patient's entire presentation. A prolonged P-R interval is not necessarily a benign finding.

BLOCK–ACCELERATION–DISSOCIATION

The next in the reclassification of A-V blocks is *block–acceleration–dissociation*. Prior to the reclassification of A-V blocks, people with EKGs like this were all labeled "third-degree block." Patients in third-degree heart block are generally presumed to have a fairly high mortality rate. But when block–acceleration–dissociation is appropriately identified, a much lower mortality rate has been noted—as long as the patients are not treated with atropine or Isuprel.

To diagnose block–acceleration–dissociation, the first thing you need is some level of A-V block. Atrial impulses are present and should be conducted to the ventricles, but they are not. There is some level of A-V block, but it doesn't fit the classic patterns of first- or second-degree block.

S5 Leads

Here's another example of the usefulness of an S5 lead.

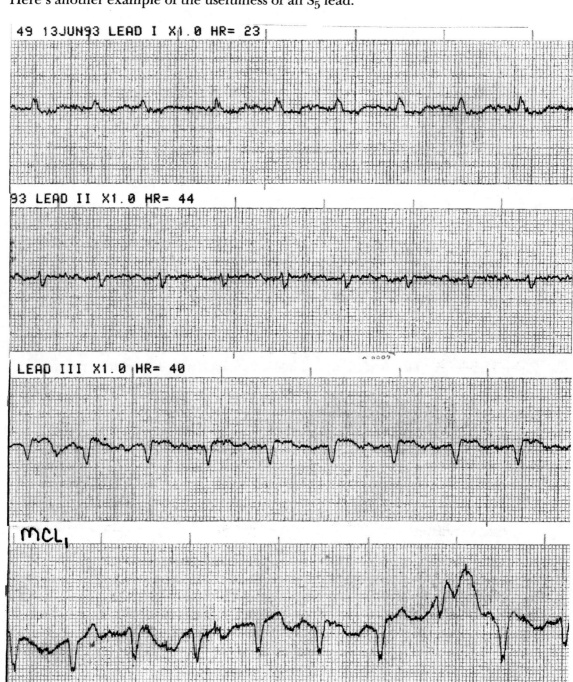

FIGURE 1.4

Figure 1.4 shows leads I, II, III, and MCL1. While in the back of the ambulance, traveling to the emergency department with a trembling patient, the paramedic had trouble deciding whether P waves were present or not. But when she ran an S5 lead, this is what she saw:

(continued on page 8)

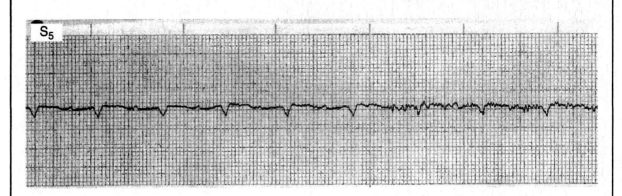

FIGURE 1.5

In Figure 1.5 you can see that there are P waves visible even though the patient continues to tremble. It takes relatively violent trembling to obscure the P waves in S$_5$. The P-R interval is constant, at about 0.22 seconds. So this is a sinus rhythm with a prolonged P-R interval.

Besides its usefulness in determining a correct diagnosis, the S$_5$ lead is also fun when you deliver your patient to the emergency department staff. Many wonder what those extra electrodes are all about!

The next thing you need is an accelerated subsidiary pacemaker. The definition we'll use for this accelerated rate is one proposed by Marriott: a rate greater than 45 per minute. The pacemaker can be either junctional or ventricular, but the rate must be greater than 45 per minute. That's one of the key differential diagnostic factors between complete heart block and block–acceleration–dissociation.

The last factor is A-V dissociation. This is when atrial and ventricular activations are separate from each other. The atrial activation does not cause the ventricular activation (or vice versa), but both are present. You'll quite frequently see "A-V dissociation" published as a diagnosis. That's like diagnosing someone as "pale." A-V dissociation is not a diagnosis. It is a description. There are at least 19 different rhythms defined, in part, by A-V dissociation. Every time you have a premature ventricular complex (PVC), you have A-V dissociation. Atrial fibrillation has A-V dissociation. And so on. A-V dissociation is only part of a description.

Rules for Block–Acceleration–Dissociation

Some level of A-V block.

Accelerated subsidiary pacemaker with a junctional or ventricular rate greater than 45 per minute.

A-V dissociation.

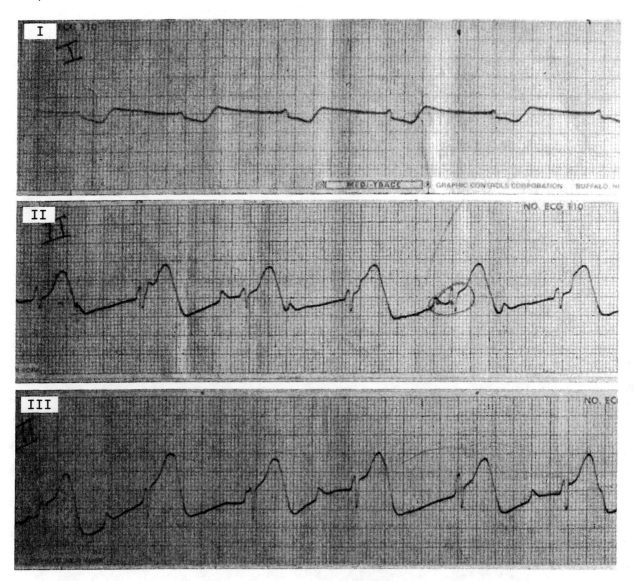

FIGURE 1.6

The patient in Figure 1.6 is a 48-year-old woman who was walking in a park during a summer fair. She experienced some nausea, vomited a couple times, had epigastric pain, mild shortness of breath, and a near-syncopal episode.

The paramedics found her to be alert and oriented to person, place, and time (AAOX3), pale, diaphoretic, and in moderate distress. She had a blood pressure of 96/50, a pulse of 56, and a respiratory rate of 24, with bilaterally clear and equal breath sounds.

The paramedics looked at her EKG (Figure 1.6) and noticed those P waves marching right on through the QRS complexes. They diagnosed her as having a "third-degree heart block" (this was in the old days). But since she was mentating well and had an adequate blood pressure, they chose not to medicate her.

What are the medications that creep into your mind every time you hear the phrase "third-degree heart block"? Atropine and Isuprel. But when do you administer atropine and Isuprel? Some people say that you give atropine and Isuprel if the patient is "symptomatic." Well, patients who are not "symptomatic" do not call 911.

What is the difference between signs and symptoms? A *symptom* is something that the patient perceives. You don't give atropine and Isuprel for something the patient perceives. You may give morphine for something the patient perceives, but not atropine or Isuprel.

Atropine and Isuprel should only be given for signs and symptoms of inadequate perfusion. Atropine and Isuprel are not given for "third-degree heart block," but for inadequate perfusion. Adequate perfusion is measured by the patient's level of consciousness and blood pressure. This patient had an adequate level of consciousness and an adequate (admittedly not great) blood pressure. We know her blood pressure was adequate because her level of consciousness was AAOX3.

So this woman received oxygen at 15 liters per minute (LPM) with a nonrebreather mask, an IV line, and a quick ride to the closest hospital. That's it. Of course, the paramedic also radioed to notify the receiving hospital that they were enroute with a 48-year-old woman in "third-degree heart block."

The staff at the receiving hospital had been to the same ACLS class as the paramedic. They wanted to properly receive this patient in third-degree heart block, so they screwed together the atropine and mixed the Isuprel drip. Upon the patient's arrival, they looked at her EKG and agreed that it was a third-degree heart block. They, however, did not share the paramedic's restraint. They decided, "Well, she's in a third-degree heart block—we gotta give atropine and Isuprel!"

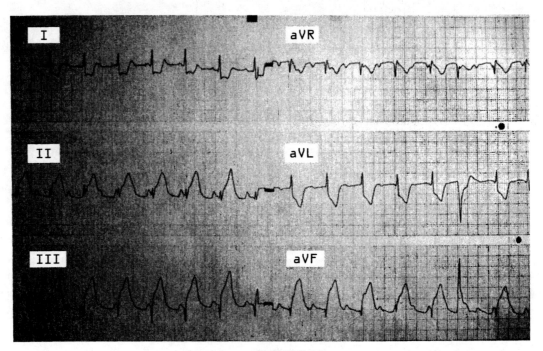

FIGURE 1.7

Atropine does not often improve the heart rate in complete heart block. But our collective habit is to give it because the protocols say so, right? Well, the emergency department staff anticipated that the atropine probably wouldn't improve this patient's heart rate. So they gave her about a milligram of atropine and then began infusing the Isuprel drip.

Figure 1.7 is the EKG obtained in the emergency department after the Isuprel drip had run for a short while. Look at the S-T elevation in lead III. What is it, about 10 or 12 millimeters? Look back at the paramedic's field strip (Figure 1.6). There, the lead III S-T elevation is only about 3 millimeters.

When you give atropine and Isuprel, you know that the drugs are doing what you want them to do if perfusion increases. Improved perfusion improves blood pressure and level of consciousness.

At the time of the paramedic's strip, the patient's mentation and blood pressure were acceptable. At the time of the emergency department's strip, her heart rate had increased from 56 to just under 100. Her S-T elevation increased also. But her blood pressure dropped to just under 70 systolic. In the next 10 minutes, her respiratory rate increased to 44, she developed fulminating pulmonary edema, and her mentation gradually decreased. In fact, she became agitated and confused to the point of being almost combative. She soon required nasotracheal intubation and was put on a ventilator with positive end expiratory pressure to manage her pulmonary edema.

Consider which medication might next be used. Of course: Dopamine. They turned on the Dopamine and gradually increased it to the point where they were delivering 20 mcg/kg/minute. It wasn't working. Then they switched to Levophed. They ran the Levophed until her urine output went to zero. They still got no increase in her blood pressure.

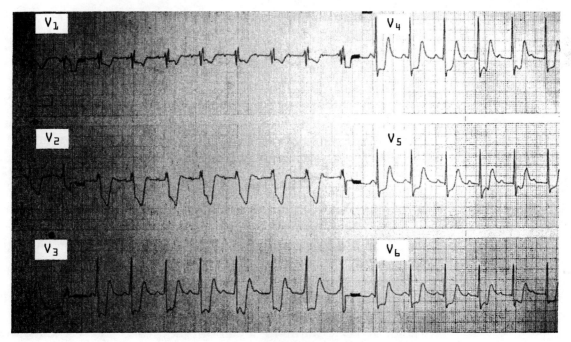

FIGURE 1.7 *continued*

So they took her to the OR and put in a balloon pump. And, of course, they put in a pacemaker because she was in "third-degree heart block."

Luckily, this woman managed to survive to hospital discharge (after a three and a half week stay). However, if she had been properly diagnosed as having block–acceleration–dissociation and left alone, she may not have had such a life-threatening experience. As it happened, the overall event left this woman a "cardiac cripple."

A cardiac cripple is someone whose life-style is dramatically impaired because his or her heart can't generate the output necessary to maintain normal function. This 48-year-old woman ended up on nasal cannula oxygen 24 hours a day, with a shoe box full of medications to take. Because she cannot tolerate the pressure caused by a firm bowel movement, she has to take stool softeners daily. And since walking to the bathroom is now too much of a strain, she requires a portable commode next to her bed.

In examining her field EKG (Figure 1.6), she does have a block of some kind. Her ventricular rate is above 45 per minute (between 54 and 60), so she has an accelerated subsidiary pacemaker. And there is dissociation between her P waves and her QRSs. The correct diagnosis of her EKG is block–acceleration–dissociation.

The final rule of block–acceleration–dissociation is this: block-acceleration-dissociation should be medicated *only* if signs of hypoperfusion exist. That's important to remember to avoid creating cardiac cripples.

Final Rule of Block–Acceleration–Dissociation

Block–acceleration–dissociation should be medicated only if signs of hypoperfusion exist.

This is an example of one of the most important reasons for the reclassification of A-V blocks. By changing the name of this classification of heart block, we can change the way we approach it. This has a huge impact on patients' collective prognoses.

For example, before 1962 there was no term for "battered child." Consequently, for years and years all kinds of battering went on and nobody did anything about it. But, in 1962, K. Henry Kempe coined the term *battered child* in a medical journal article, and all of a sudden things changed.[2] Programs were developed, and child abuse became illegal. Soon after this, the term *battered women* came into use, followed by the development of programs and legislation. Much of this occurred because someone finally came up with a name for the situation.

With the reclassification name of block–acceleration–dissociation, we should be able to prevent the management errors that go along with over-diagnosis of "third-degree heart block."

Now, a lot of people have not learned the labels associated with Marriott's reclassification of A-V blocks. And you may be thinking, "If I call in to notify a receiving hospital that I'm bringing in a 48-year-old woman in block–acceleration–dissociation, they won't know what I'm talking about!" Well, that's okay. Because they certainly won't be screwing together the atropine or mixing up a bag of D_5W and Isuprel while you're on your way in. And maybe the unfamiliar label will cause them to take the time to evaluate the *patient* before responding to a "third-degree heart block" in the manner that many have before.

Some people ask me what course of treatment, in my opinion, would have been more appropriate for this patient. It's difficult to play "Monday morning quarterback" on this (or any) case. First, you have to understand that this case occurred prior to the advent of thrombolytic therapy. Considering that, this patient could have first been given a small fluid challenge. If her blood pressure increased to a safe level, they could have achieved pain control by using nitrates or some morphine. And then they could have admitted her to the CCU to rest and watch uninteresting soap operas for a few days. Perhaps, then, she could have been discharged healthy, without any other pharmacologic intervention.

Given today's pharmacology, she would probably have been a candidate for getting TPA, streptokinase, or another of those wonderful clot-busting drugs to treat her inferior wall myocardial infarction.

OCCASIONAL DROPPED BEATS: TYPE I AND TYPE II

The next of the reclassifications of A-V blocks is similar to second-degree heart block. It is called *occasional dropped beats* and is divided into two groups: *type I* and *type II*.

Occasional Dropped Beats Type I (Wenckebach)

The first group, occasional dropped beats type I, was originally called Wenckebach and later called Mobitz I. The EKG shows consecutive atrial impulses preceding progressively lengthening P-R intervals, until the non-conducted or "dropped" beat.

This guy, Wenckebach, was a pretty spectacular physician in my estimation. He was able to describe the Wenckebach pattern in 1899. The reason I find that so impressive is that the electrocardiogram wasn't developed until 1903![1] By listening to the patient's apical pulse with his stethoscope, while looking at the patient's jugular veins, he was able to describe this particular phenomenon without the benefit of an electrocardiogram.

Observing the P-R intervals lengthening until a beat is dropped is the way most of us were taught to recognize this rhythm. And in the "pure" Wenckebach, even the shortest P-R interval is usually longer than 0.20 seconds with a QRS complex that is usually within normal limits. This indicates the absence of a bundle branch block.

But there is another technique you can use to recognize a Wenckebach rhythm. When you first look at a Wenckebach on the EKG, you should notice that there are groups of beats. Then, if you look at the R to R interval (R-R interval) instead of the P-R interval, you will notice that the R-R interval progressively *shortens* prior to the dropped QRS complex.

In addition to this, the longest R-R interval (the one that contains the dropped ventricular impulse) is less than two times the length of the short-est R-R interval. I know that seems like a lot to think about, but keep read-ing. It will make sense soon.

Rules for Occasional Dropped Beats: Type I (Wenckebach)

Groups of beats.

Consecutive atrial impulses preceding progressively lengthening P-R intervals prior to a nonconducted atrial impulse (a "dropped" QRS complex).

R-R interval progressively shortens prior to the "dropped" QRS complex.

The shortest P-R interval is usually longer than 0.20 seconds.

The longest R-R interval is less than two times the length of the shortest R-R interval. (The longest R-R interval is the one that contains the dropped QRS complex.)

The QRS complex is usually within normal limits.

When you were taught to read EKGs, you were probably taught to look first at P waves, right? This is because early EKG teachers established the bad habit of teaching information from the "top" of the heart "down." First you learn about P waves, then you learn about sinus arrhythmia, then atrial fibrillation, atrial flutter, and so on. Then you learned about junc-tional rhythms, and somewhere toward the end of the class you learned about ventricular rhythms.

What's going to kill the patient first? Ventricular arrhythmias. So, when I teach a basic EKG class, I start out with ventricular rhythms. This throws people off. They might even search for a textbook that uses this same progression of instruction. There hasn't been one—until now! But at least it gets people to focus on what's important about any EKG, and that is the QRS complex!

The QRS complex most directly correlates to how well your patient's heart is functioning. What I encourage is this: When you first look at an EKG, rather than sticking it up to your nose and looking for P waves, hold it away from you, at arm's length. Look at the QRS complexes and try to get an overall feel for the strip.

When you do this, you'll notice whether there are grouped beats. When you notice grouped beats, occasional dropped beats type I should spring to mind. Then you need to look closer to determine whether you've got it or not. If you can see the P-R intervals getting progressively longer before you come upon a dropped beat, you've got an easy one. If not, there is another way.

Look at the QRS complexes. In occasional dropped beats type I the R-R intervals become progressively shorter until a dropped beat occurs.

And if you take the longest R-R interval (the one including the nonconducted atrial impulse), it is shorter than two times the length of the shortest R-R interval.

Let's start with this strip.

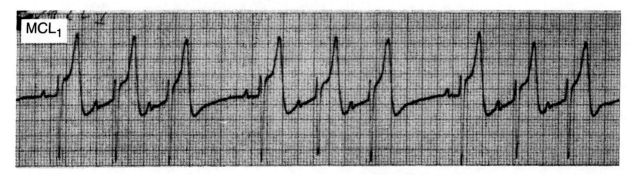

FIGURE 1.8

Figure 1.8 is an MCL$_1$ strip from a patient with an anterior wall myocardial infarction. Each P-R interval gets a little bit longer, until one of the P waves doesn't conduct to the ventricles. Do you see the nonconducted P wave perched on top of the T wave?

This is a fairly simple to spot occasional dropped beats type I, or Wenckebach. But do you also see how you can notice groups of three beats? Take a look at each group; the R-R intervals become progressively shorter. And two times the shortest R-R interval is longer than the R-R interval that contains the dropped P wave.

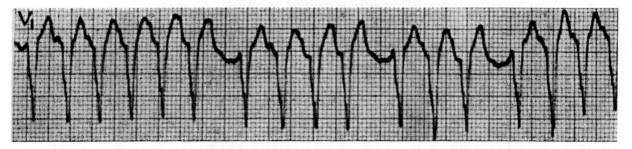

FIGURE 1.9 (Reproduced by permission of Dr. Henry J. L. Marriott, Director of Clinical Research and Education, Rogers Heart Foundation, St. Anthony's Hospital, St. Petersburg, Florida.)

In Figure 1.9, you may have difficulty finding P waves.[*] But look at what's happening to the R-R intervals. They get progressively shorter until a long one starts a new group. The longest R-R interval is shorter than two

---

[*]People who are into P waves can find P waves anywhere. You can put an electroencephalogram in front of them, and they will show you where the P waves are. Marriott calls this the "P preoccupation syndrome." So, if you're really into it, you can probably find a P wave or two in Figure 1.9.

times the shortest R-R. So you've just diagnosed a type I occasional dropped beats (Wenckebach), without a visible P-R interval.

Anatomically speaking, a type I occasional dropped beats block (Wenckebach) occurs in the A-V node and is usually benign. It usually doesn't cause serious problems for patients, especially in the prehospital setting. If they get bradycardic and hypoperfused, a little gentle atropine is often all it takes to improve their perfusion.

Recently, however, it has come to light that patients with an ischemic cardiac event who survive to be discharged from the hospital and who are still in occasional dropped beats-type blocks upon discharge may have a different long-term prognosis. It has been suggested that patients with type I block who did *not* get a permanent pacemaker implanted during the course of their treatment may have a slightly higher morbidity ratio than their counterparts with type II block (who receive pacemakers). There has not yet been enough research to confirm this one way or another. But there remains a strong suspicion that occasional dropped beats type I heart block may not be as benign a diagnosis upon discharge as it is upon admission.

So, even though type I heart block patients are still considered to have a relatively benign heart block (especially in the emergent prehospital phases), researchers are beginning to wonder. They're beginning to think that, for long-term management, patients who remain in a type I heart block after the course of their infarction should perhaps receive a pacemaker. Of course, people who demonstrate a type II heart block continue to get a pacemaker right away!

Occasional Dropped Beats Type II

Occasional dropped beats type II is when you have consecutive atrial impulses conducted with a constant P-R interval prior to a nonconducted atrial impulse (a "dropped" QRS complex). This was also first described by Wenckebach, in 1906.[1] In 1924, Mobitz confirmed all of Wenckebach's work on the two types of occasional dropped beats heart blocks. They were then (immodestly!) renamed Mobitz type I and Mobitz type II A-V heart blocks.[1]

If I had my way, I would give credit to the founder, the person who did all the clinical work and truly first discovered these heart blocks. I would rename them Wenckebach type I and Wenckebach type II. But I guess we can't have everything.

The anatomical difference between type I and type II occasional dropped beats is this: type I is a block located in the A-V node and is usually benign; type II blocks are infranodal, located within the bundle branches, and are always malignant. This is why type II heart blocks are strong indications for a pacemaker.

In a "pure" type II occasional dropped beats heart block, the P-R interval is usually normal, between 0.12 and 0.20 seconds. But there is a bundle branch block present, evidenced by the QRS complex measuring greater than 0.12 seconds.

Basically, occasional dropped beats type II indicates a *fixed* block in one bundle branch and an *intermittent* block in the other bundle branch.

We were called for a 58-year-old male who complained of dizziness after sneezing. He hadn't seen a doctor in the last 20 years and wasn't interested in seeing one this day. Somebody else had called "the damn ambulance," he hadn't, and he didn't plan on going anywhere in it. So I offered, "Hey, as long as we're here, why don't I give you a free blood pressure check and electrocardiogram?"

"Sure, you kids do whatever you want."

Rules for Occasional Dropped Beats: Type II

Consecutive atrial impulses conducted with a constant P-R interval prior to a nonconducted atrial impulse (a "dropped" QRS complex).

Usually a normal P-R interval; between 0.12 and 0.20 seconds.

A bundle branch block; the QRS complex measures greater than 0.12 seconds.

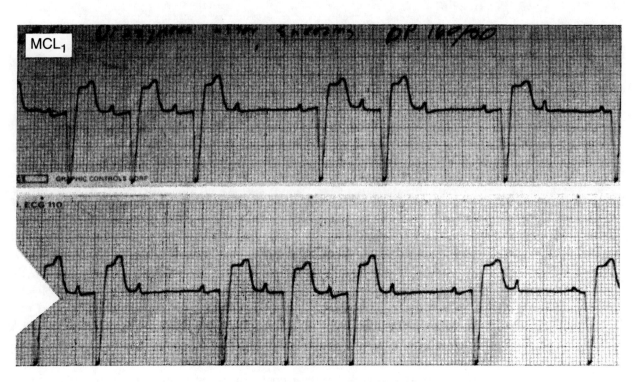

FIGURE 1.10a

Figure 1.10a is his MCL$_1$ strip. You might notice grouped beats here, and that's good. But when you try to apply the rules for Wenckebach, they don't fit. The R-R intervals are exactly the same prior to the dropped cycle. And two times the shortest one is exactly the same as the longest R-R interval (the one containing the nonconducted atrial impulse). It doesn't fit occasional dropped beats type I (Wenckebach).

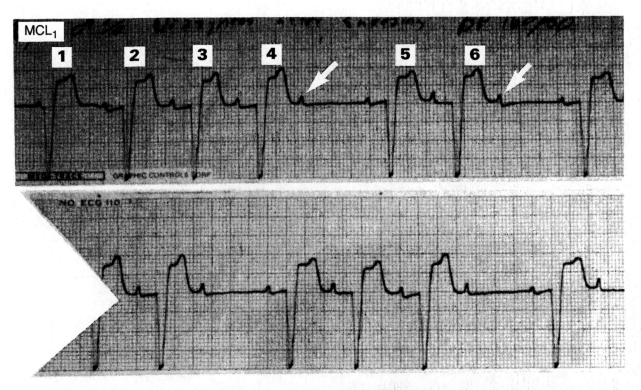

FIGURE 1.10b

So we have consecutive atrial impulses conducted with a constant P-R interval of less than 0.20 seconds prior to the dropped cycle. And this patient has a QRS complex greater than 0.12 seconds. He has a left bundle branch block (you'll learn in Chapter Two how to diagnose left from right bundle branch block). This is occasional dropped beats type II.

In this patient's case, as you can see in Figure 1.10b, the left bundle branch has a fixed block and the right bundle branch has an intermittent block. The sinus impulse fires, conducts down the right bundle branch, and fires the ventricles, producing QRS complex number 1. Because the left bundle branch is blocked, the QRS is wider than 0.12 seconds. The same thing happens to produce QRS complex number 2; the sinus impulse travels down the right bundle branch and fires the ventricles to produce QRS number 2. QRS complexes numbers 3 and 4 are fired the same way. But the next atrial impulse finds the right bundle branch blocked also, and thus it is unable to fire the ventricles (arrow). This produces a "dropped," nonconducted atrial beat. Because the right bundle branch block is only intermittent, the cycle begins again as soon as the right bundle branch is no longer blocked. QRS complexes numbers 5 and 6 are produced by sinus impulses conducting down the right bundle branch. And then the next sinus impulse finds the right bundle branch blocked (arrow). And so on.

Type II occasional dropped beats heart block is bad news. It is considered malignant and indicates the need for a pacemaker. Who is to say how long that intermittent right bundle branch block is going to remain intermittent? If it becomes a *fixed* right bundle branch block, the patient will then have a complete heart block.

Those who have the capability to apply an external pacemaker to patients should hook it up to this sort of patient. Put the pacer patches on and attach the cables without turning on the machine. If the patient's intermittent bundle branch block becomes a fixed bundle branch block, followed by a drop in the heart rate and perfusion, then they can turn the pacer on.

2:1 BLOCK TYPE I AND TYPE II

The next in the reclassification of A-V blocks is *2:1 block*. 2:1 block is also divided into *type I* and *type II*. This is another heart block that has classically been overdiagnosed (as "second-degree type II") and consequently overtreated.

A 2:1 block is when you have two atrial impulses for every QRS complex. One atrial impulse is conducted, the next one is not. The next impulse is conducted, the next one is not. And so on.

Many EKG classes and workbooks state that, in the face of 2:1 A-V conduction, it is *impossible* to determine type I from type II block. Well, we will now show you how to recognize 2:1 type I from 2:1 type II heart blocks.

Traditionally, 2:1 block has always been considered a type II second-degree heart block. In reality, a large percentage of 2:1 heart blocks may actually be type I. As discussed, type II heart blocks are strong indications for a pacemaker. So, theoretically, if we consider every 2:1 block a type II heart block, we end up with lots of people implanted with pacemakers they may not need. In any case, you *can* differentiate between them!

2:1 Block Type I

In 2:1 block type I, the P-R interval is greater than 0.20 seconds and the QRS complex is less than 0.12 seconds. This means there is a prolonged P-R interval *and* an absence of bundle branch block. This goes along with the same anatomic and prognostic correlations as occasional dropped beats type I; 2:1 block type I is in the A-V node and considered to be benign.

2:1 Block Type II

Type II 2:1 block is just the opposite. The P-R interval is within normal limits (0.12 to 0.20 seconds). And the QRS complex is wide (measuring greater than 0.12 seconds), indicating the presence of a bundle branch block. 2:1 block type II is an infranodal block, is considered malignant, and is a strong indication for a pacemaker.

Of course, everyone likes to play "What if?" What if you have a 2:1 block with a prolonged P-R interval *and* a bundle branch block? The key factor is the wide QRS complex, indicating the presence of an infranodal block. If you have a 2:1 block with a prolonged P-R interval and a bundle branch block, consider it to be a type II 2:1 block.

Figure 1.11 is an MCL_1 strip, but before we discuss this rhythm, does this look like a "normal" MCL_1 strip? Some of you may be thinking that, since you don't often look at MCL_1 strips (at least not before reading this book), you can only say that it looks familiar. Well, it might look familiar to lead II electrocardiologists because it has upright QRS complexes. Upright QRS complexes are normal in lead II, but not in MCL_1. In MCL_1 the QRS complexes are normally negative. You'll see that statement again when we get to the chapter about infarct identification, Chapter Eleven. The upright QRS complex and the little bit of S-T depression in MCL_1 indicate that this patient is having a posterior wall myocardial infarction.

2:1 Block

Rules for 2:1 Block Type I	Rules for 2:1 Block Type II
Two atrial impulses for every QRS complex.	Two atrial impulses for every QRS complex.
A prolonged P-R interval (greater than 0.20 seconds).	A normal P-R interval (0.12 to 0.20 seconds).
A QRS within normal limits (less than 0.12 seconds).	A wide QRS (greater than 0.12 seconds); a bundle branch block.

If you have a 2:1 block with a prolonged P-R interval *and* a bundle branch block, consider it to be a type II.

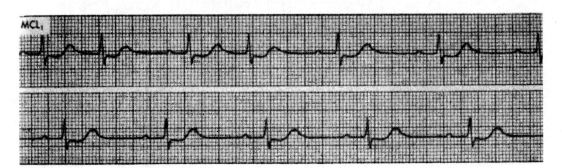

FIGURE 1.11 (Henry J. L. Marriott and M. Boudreau Conover, *Advanced Concepts in Arrhythmias*, 2nd ed., 1989; C. V. Mosby, St. Louis, MO.)

The patient in Figure 1.11 started out in a classic Wenckebach pattern, or occasional dropped beats type I. You can see a P wave with a long P-R interval; the next P wave is on top of the T wave and precedes a longer P-R interval; and the next T wave has a P wave on its proximal side that is not conducted to the ventricles.

I admit that the dropped P wave is somewhat hard to see. Look at the last half of the previous T wave. Do you see how smooth it is? But the last half of the next T wave has a pimple on it. One of my two T wave rules, is this: "Teenagers have pimples, T waves do not."

Given this pattern of a long P-R interval, a longer P-R interval, and then a dropped atrial impulse, we have occasional dropped beats type I, or Wenckebach.

But then something changes. The patient's overall rate slows. There is a P wave for every QRS complex, and every T wave has a pimple. Okay, I agree with you. If I hadn't seen the earlier section of strip where there were smooth T waves, I wouldn't have been able to recognize that pimple as being a P wave on a T wave. I would not have known that this particular strip was a 2:1 block. But, luckily, I did see the earlier section of strip and could then easily recognize the 2:1 A-V block.

When you want to differentiate type I from type II 2:1 block, look at the conducted beats. In Figure 1.11, the P-R interval is 0.24 seconds, and the QRS complex is 0.07 seconds wide. Prolonged P-R interval, normal QRS complex, one dropped beat. This is a 2:1 block type I, or a 2:1 Wenckebach.

Before this differentiation, people would say, "Oh, this guy was in a Wenckebach and then he changed into a type II!" It may happen, but it's very unusual. If you can find an EKG strip where the patient goes from a Wenckebach or occasional dropped beats type I heart block into a type II heart block, I'll pay you money for it. I will pay $100.00 cash to the person who can bring me such a strip.

What has changed here (Figure 1.11) is the conduction ratio. It changed from 3:2 conduction to 2:1 conduction. The type of block is the same—no better, no worse. There's just been a change in the conduction ratio. If this patient is hypoperfusing due to this lower rate, a little gentle atropine is likely to bring the rate right back up to par.

About now, you are probably asking yourself, "What does he mean? Why does he keep saying 'gentle atropine'?" When I went to paramedic school, atropine was one of the few medications we were taught to give *IV push*. That meant to stick the needle in the injection site and give the plunger one quick, healthy push before opening up the line and flushing it in. In fact, we were taught that if we gave atropine *slow* IV push it could cause "reflex bradycardia."

Have you ever seen reflex bradycardia secondary to giving atropine? I'm sure there are a few documented cases of it. But I have seen more cases of ventricular tachycardia and ventricular fibrillation from when atropine is administered too rapidly.

Very seldom do medications need to be given quickly. Electricity needs to be given quickly. Medications usually do not. A great example is D_{50}. It's considered a benign drug—not a dangerous drug to give unless you blow up a vein, right? So you crimp off the line to give the D_{50} and, especially if you used a small angiocath, you really have to crank on that plunger to inject the dextrose. Well, even with a wide-bore angiocath, dextrose in a 50% concentration is corrosive to the inside of a vein!

I have a friend with a seizure disorder. Every time he has received D_{50}, he has ended up with thrombophlebitis from the IV site all the way up to his subclavian vein! Thrombophlebitis is not a pleasant experience. But if you give medications such as D_{50} slowly, gently, allowing them to dilute in the blood, you won't cause this kind of problem.

Anesthesiologists and the people who run progressive cardiology units give atropine slowly. They also may give the patient a dose of only 0.2

or 0.3 mg. This is what I mean by "gentle atropine": give it slowly and stop administration when the desired effect begins to occur. I am not trying to change your protocols. I can't do that anyway. I just happen to know that a lot of people who are very good and very experienced in cardiology are giving low, slow doses of atropine, just enough to gently raise the heart rate and obtain better perfusion.

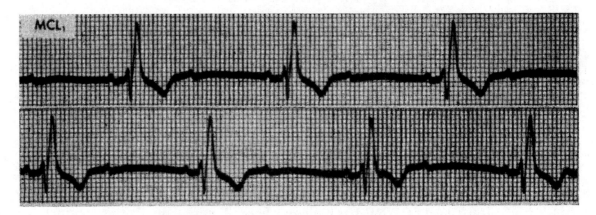

FIGURE 1.12 (Henry J. L. Marriott and M. Boudreau Conover, *Advanced Concepts in Arrhythmias*, 2nd ed., 1989; C. V. Mosby, St. Louis, MO.)

In Figure 1.12 you can see two P waves for each QRS complex. This is a 2:1 block. The P-R interval for the conducted beat is 0.16 seconds. If you look at the QRS complex you can see that it's wide, about 0.13 seconds. This happens to be a right bundle branch block pattern. So Figure 1.12 shows an EKG rhythm that is a 2:1 block and has a normal P-R interval and a wide QRS complex. This is 2:1 block type II. This patient needs a pacemaker.

This patient needs a pacemaker because he has a fixed right bundle branch block and an intermittent left bundle branch block. The fixed right bundle branch block is creating the wide QRS complex. The conducted P wave travels down the left bundle branch and activates the ventricles. The dropped P wave is not conducted when the left bundle branch becomes blocked. The next P wave finds the left bundle branch conducting again. The next P wave finds it blocked. And what happens if the left bundle branch stays blocked? The patient will then be in complete heart block.

2:1 block type II is infranodal, considered malignant, and is a strong indication for a pacemaker.

HIGH-GRADE A-V BLOCK TYPE I AND TYPE II

High-grade A-V block is the next in the reclassification of A-V blocks and also is divided into *type I* and *type II*. High-grade A-V block is when there are at least two consecutive atrial impulses that fail to be conducted to the ventricles.

Remember the first rule of occasional dropped beats: there are at least two consecutive atrial impulses that are conducted to the ventricles. High-grade A-V block is when at least two consecutive atrial impulses are *not* conducted. There is at least one episode of 3:1 conduction.

According to Marriott, this should *only* be considered a "block" in the presence of reasonable atrial rates of 135/minute or less. There's no significant "magic" to that rate limit of 135. It's just what is considered reasonable. If the atrial rate was 250, you would *expect* to find nonconducted atrial impulses. Thus, that would not be a block.

To differentiate between type I and type II high-grade A-V block, as with 2:1 A-V block type I and type II, look at the conducted cycles. High-grade A-V block type I has a prolonged P-R interval (greater than 0.20 seconds) and a narrow QRS complex (less than 0.12 seconds). High-grade A-V block type II has a normal P-R interval (0.12 to 0.20 seconds) and a wide QRS complex (greater than 0.12 seconds), indicating the presence of a bundle branch block.

Rules for High-Grade A-V Block

At least two consecutive atrial impulses fail to be conducted to the ventricles.

Reasonable atrial rates (135/minute or less).

High-Grade A-V Block

TYPE I

A prolonged P-R interval (greater than 0.20 seconds).

A QRS within normal limits (less than 0.12 seconds).

TYPE II

A normal P-R interval (0.12 to 0.20 seconds).

A wide QRS (greater than 0.12 seconds); a bundle branch block.

If you have a high-grade A-V block with a prolonged P-R interval *and* a bundle branch block, consider it to be a type II.

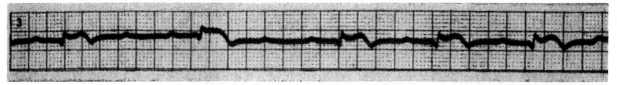

FIGURE 1.13 (Henry J. L. Marriott and M. Boudreau Conover, *Advanced Concepts in Arrhythmias*, 2nd ed., 1989; C. V. Mosby, St. Louis, MO.)

Figure 1.13 is a lead III EKG strip. If you map out the P waves, you can see that there is a P wave hidden in each T wave. And there are two instances when two P waves do not conduct to the ventricles. In those cases, only the third P wave produces a QRS complex. Therefore, this is occasionally a high-grade A-V block.

Now look at the conducted complexes. There is a long P-R interval, about 0.30 seconds. And the QRS complex is narrow, about 0.04 or 0.05 seconds. That makes this a high-grade A-V block type I.

This particular patient also has a small q wave with a little S-T elevation and a flipped T wave. This is probably an inferior wall infarction. I say that because inferior wall infarctions tend to go along with type I heart blocks. Or, perhaps, type I heart blocks tend to go along with inferior wall infarctions. In any case, inferior MIs are commonly associated with all type I heart blocks.

The way to treat any poor perfusion due to this slow rate is with a little gentle atropine.

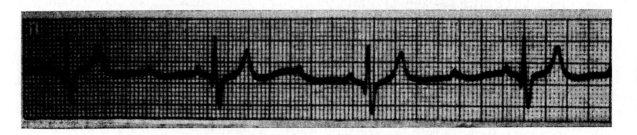

FIGURE 1.14   (Henry J. L. Marriott and M. Boudreau Conover, *Advanced Concepts in Arrhythmias,* 2nd ed., 1989; C. V. Mosby, St. Louis, MO.)

This particular patient (Figure 1.14) had syncopal episodes related to a cardiac arrhythmia. In this patient's lead I, you can map out the P waves and see that each T wave has a hidden P wave that does not conduct to the ventricles. This hidden, nonconductive P wave is followed by another P wave that does not conduct. But every third P wave conducts. This demonstrates a constant 3:1 conduction ratio; this is a high-grade A-V block.

Looking at the conducted impulse, you can see a P-R interval of about 0.14 or 0.16 seconds. It's well within the normal limits for a P-R interval. But the QRS complex is wide. It's about 0.12 seconds. Any supraventricular complex that is 0.12 seconds wide or wider has a bundle branch block.

Figure 1.14 is a high-grade A-V block type II. This patient needs a pacemaker. This patient's heart is beating only because every third impulse is able to conduct down one bundle branch (the left bundle branch). All the other impulses find both bundle branches blocked. This patient is just a "hair's breadth" away from complete heart block—or from being in ventricular asystole with only nonconducted P waves present. If an external pacemaker is available, have it in place and ready to function in the event that the patient stops conducting every third P wave while in your care.

When you're making a destination decision regarding this patient, you must consider this patient's need for a pacemaker. If Our Lady of Great Goodness hospital and Hard Rock Memorial hospital are within similar distance, but Hard Rock Memorial can quickly put in a pacemaker while Our Lady of Great Goodness cannot, take the patient to Hard Rock Memorial. This patient needs a pacemaker, pronto!

COMPLETE HEART BLOCK

Formerly called "third-degree heart block," the next in the reclassification of A-V blocks is *complete heart block*. Complete heart block can be divided into *junctional* or *ventricular* categories, depending upon the location of the escape pacemaker. Some people call them *proximal* or *distal* complete heart block.

Most junctional complete heart blocks are due to a structural deficit caused by calcification of the aortic valve, degenerative diseases of the cardiac skeleton, or the like. However, the majority of complete heart blocks have a ventricular escape mechanism (when the pacemaker that fires the ventricles is located in the His–Purkinje system or the ventricles). So ventricular complete heart blocks are the ones you'll most likely see in the myocardial infarction setting.

The first element in diagnosis of complete heart block is that there can be no A-V conduction. Absolutely *no* atrial impulses conduct through to the ventricles.

The second requirement is that there must be *plenty* of atrial impulses present. Atrial impulses consist of P waves, atrial fibrillation, or atrial flutter. So there are plenty of atrial impulses present, but no A-V conduction.

The final requirement for a diagnosis of complete heart block is a *slow* junctional or ventricular escape rate of less than 45 per minute. This is how you gain a differential diagnosis between block–acceleration–dissociation and complete heart block. If the ventricular rate is greater than 45 per minute, the diagnosis is block–acceleration–dissociation and the patient should *not* be medicated (unless signs or symptoms of hypoperfusion exist). If the ventricular rate is less than 45 per minute and the patient is showing signs of hypoperfusion, appropriate treatment includes a pacemaker.

According to Marriott, in order to diagnose complete heart block, "it is complete only when the opportunity for conduction is optimal, yet none occurs." You must have plenty of atrial impulses that should be conducting, but do not. If you have no atrial impulses, then there is nothing to be blocked. So that situation cannot be called a block.

Rules for Complete Heart Block

No A-V conduction.

Plenty of atrial impulses.

A junctional or ventricular rate of less than 45 per minute.

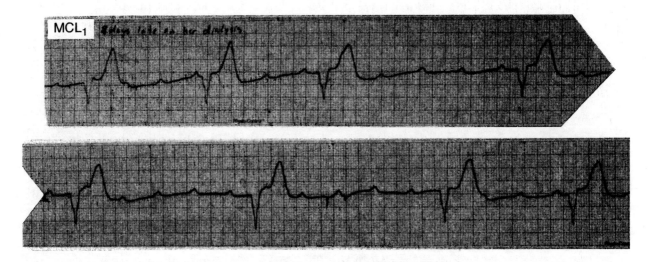

FIGURE 1.15

As Marriott says, it's sort of like diagnosing absolute fidelity. Many of us remain "fidel" only because the opportunity to be "infidel" has not been optimal. In order to be diagnosed as having absolute fidelity, you need to be locked in a well-stocked hotel suite for 48 hours with an attractive—and assertive—member of your sexual preference. If, at the end of 48 hours, you emerge victorious against temptation, the diagnosis of absolute fidelity may be applied.

Looking at Figure 1.15, what catches your attention first? Hopefully, the rate. It's slow. It's *really* slow! There is a wide ventricular escape at a rate of about 20 per minute. And there are lots of P waves. What QRS could resist all those alluring little P waves, I ask you? Finally, you can see that there is no A-V conduction. This is complete heart block.

There is a slight irregularity to the ventricular pacemaker. It may confuse some people into thinking that there are some conducted beats. However, the differing P-R intervals testify to the lack of A-V conduction. The escape pacemaker simply happens to be firing irregularly. There is no law written anywhere that says pacemakers *have* to fire regularly!

Do you notice anything else striking about Figure 1.15? How about those seriously big T waves? This patient is a 42-year-old woman who was suicidally depressed because of being turned down for a kidney transplant. She had been on dialysis three days a week for a year and a half and decided to commit suicide by not going to dialysis. She hadn't been to dialysis in 8 days. And she'd been eating a lot of cantaloupe. She must have learned that, although bananas have an average content of 450 milligrams of potassium, cantaloupes contain 1700 milligrams of potassium. Therefore, she tried to quicken her demise by eating cantaloupe.

What's the normal blood level of potassium? It's 3.5 to 5 (or 5.5, depending on which institution you're in). Her potassium was 9.6. For most of us, this would be a fatal potassium level. Dialysis patients, however, develop a higher tolerance to potassium levels, so she wasn't dead yet.

Back to her T waves. These tall, pointy T waves should catch your attention no matter what rhythm they are associated with. This brings us to the second of my two T wave rules: "If the T wave looks like it would hurt your butt if you sat on it, the patient is probably hyperkalemic." That's the rule of hyperkalemic T waves.

Taigman's T-Wave Rules

Rule 1: Teenagers have pimples, T waves do not.

Rule 2: If the T waves look like they would hurt your butt if you sat on them, the patient is probably hyperkalemic.

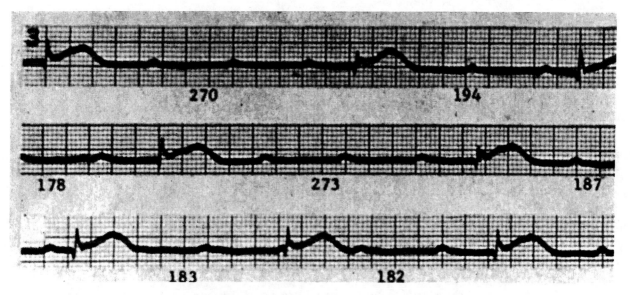

FIGURE 1.16 (Reproduced by permission of Dr. Henry J. L. Marriott, Director of Clinical Research and Education, Rogers Heart Foundation, St. Anthony's Hospital, St. Petersburg, Florida.)

Figure 1.16 is an EKG strip from an infant with congenital heart disease. This EKG has a very slow rate, lots of P waves, and no A-V conduction. Notice the very narrow QRS complex. This is a junctional (or proximal) complete heart block.

Complete heart block is considered the ultimate indication for a pacemaker. In the prehospital setting, an infant that presents with this kind of EKG strip is probably having some kind of pacemaker failure. That's because these kids tend to have pacemakers installed as soon as the anomaly is discovered—usually soon after delivery and before they leave the hospital.

Okay. Figure 1.17 shows another one of those strips that I simply have to share. Often, when this kind of rhythm is displayed on your monitor, your radio report includes the comment, "Our EKG equipment is malfunctioning and we can't get a clear tracing. We'll show you when we get there!"

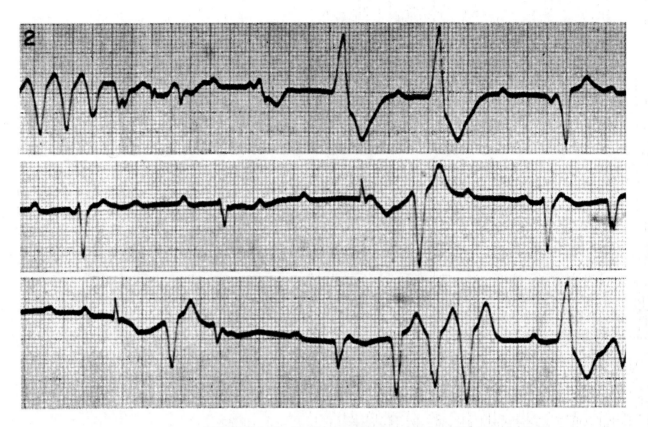

FIGURE 1.17 (Reproduced by permission of Dr. Henry J. L. Marriott, Director of Clinical Research and Education, Rogers Heart Foundation, St. Anthony's Hospital, St. Petersburg, Florida.)

What do you see in Figure 1.17? It looks like some runs of ventricular tachycardia with an underlying complete heart block. Complete heart block with ventricular tachycardia...hm-m-m. Let's divide them into separate entities, shall we?

With complete heart block, what drugs come to mind? Atropine, Isuprel, and epinephrine. What drugs come to mind for ventricular tachycardia? Lidocaine and Bretylium.

Most of us have taken the ACLS class. When they run the mega-code and you've got a patient in complete heart block, you give them atropine. That doesn't work, so you start the Isuprel drip. Then the mega-code instructor starts to hit the little button on the arrhythmia simulator that makes PVCs. What's the first thing you're supposed to do when you see the PVCs? Turn off the Isuprel. Why? Because Isuprel can cause ventricular tachycardia. So Isuprel is contraindicated in patients with ventricular tachycardia. So is atropine. The drug of choice in ventricular tachycardia is lidocaine. But in what setting is lidocaine absolutely contraindicated? Complete heart block. So Figure 1.17 presents quite a problem. Well, think about it. If you had everything available to you, if you were in the middle of a coronary care unit, what would be the optimal way to treat this patient? The answer: put in a pacemaker first. Once your pacemaker is capturing, *then* give the lidocaine!

But in a place where you don't have a pacemaker available, it's kind of a crap shoot. There are no good options. If you give atropine, there's a small chance that you may speed up the underlying rhythm and wipe out the ventricular ectopy. If you give lidocaine first, there's a very small chance that you'll wipe out the ectopy and increase the conduction of the underlying rhythm. There is also a good chance that either of these approaches will result in cardiac arrest.

Or, you could do nothing. That's hard to do, isn't it? We're usually the kind of people who like to *do* things. To do *nothing* would be difficult for most of us. But one of the first things taught any medical practitioner is to *do no harm*.

Without a pacemaker, I'm not convinced that we can safely medicate this patient without making the situation worse. Some people may suggest Bretylium. But a patient with this rhythm is quite likely to be hypotensive and thus suffering from hypoperfusion. I'd be very concerned about giving Bretylium to a hypotensive patient. Instead, I'd be most inclined to treat this patient with an accelerator. My *vehicle* accelerator! Yes, there are still medical patients whose problems are best handled by a quick ride to the hospital.

Okay. Time for another case study.

We were called to a low-income apartment complex on a "sick case." As we walked up to the door, we were greeted by a fairly well known local prostitute. I'd taken care of her on numerous occasions after assaults, when she was found drunk and unconscious in the street, and for various fulminating pelvic inflammatory diseases. She pointed us toward the bathroom and said, "That (censored) has been in there puking for an hour! I would like you to get his (censored) out of my bathroom, 'cause I've got to pee!"

She had dialed 911, with the chief complaint of having to pee.

As we walked back to see this guy, she told us that he'd consumed a quart of Jack Daniels in about a 10-minute period and had been puking ever since. We found him draped over the commode, noting that he had been incontinent of both urine and feces. He also was covered with emesis because he only occasionally managed to hit the toilet. The scene had a significantly nasty olfactory element.

There was no light in the bathroom (of course), so we pulled him out into the living room and asked, "What's going on?" He greeted us with some terrifically slurred utterances that sounded as though they were probably rude. Mostly, he was doing a lot of moaning and didn't seem to be very well oriented (as you might imagine). He was drenched in sweat and cold to the touch, even through double gloves. We weren't surprised that he had no blood pressure, especially after finding his carotid pulse to be weak.

After providing him with some oxygen, we hooked him up to the cardiac monitor. Figure 1.18 is his EKG, leads I, II, III, and MCL$_1$.

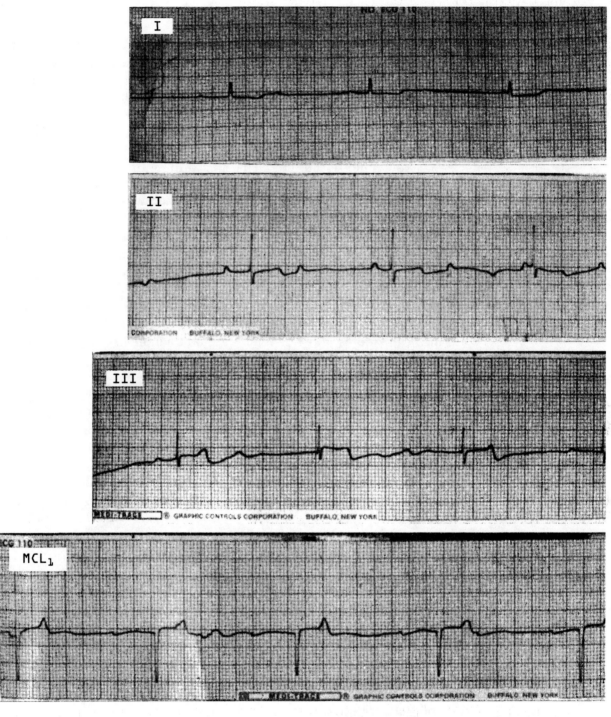

FIGURE 1.18

As you can see, he has a ventricular rate of about 40 and P waves marching right on through the QRS complexes. He has a ventricular rate less than 45, he has lots of atrial impulses, and no A-V conduction. So this gentleman's EKG is complete heart block with narrow QRS complexes.

We started an IV and gave him half a milligram of atropine. It didn't change anything. Gave him another half-milligram of atropine. Didn't change anything. Gave him a full milligram of atropine and his pupils dilated. Still no change in the heart rate or perfusion. At that point we headed for the ambulance with him. Once there, what do you suppose was the next medication we administered? Most people might proceed to an Isuprel drip. But not me. I don't think Isuprel is very beneficial.

How does Isuprel work? It's pure beta. Beta increases the heart rate and force of myocardial contraction, increasing myocardial oxygen demand. Beta also dilates the peripheral vasculature. So, on one hand, Isuprel attempts to increase perfusion by increasing the rate and force of myocardial contraction. But, at the same time, it decreases perfusion by dilating peripheral vasculature (lowering blood pressure). So, in order for Isuprel to improve the patient's overall perfusion, the heart rate must be increased further and faster than the peripheral vasculature is being dilated. When you give Isuprel to increase perfusion in bradycardia refractory to atropine, you may compound the original problem with its side effects. This causes an additional workload on an already malfunctioning heart. That doesn't strike me as being a smart thing to do.

Have you ever used an epinephrine drip? Think about it. What is the difference between epinephrine and Isuprel? Epinephrine has beta *and* alpha properties. Its beta properties increase heart rate and the force of myocardial contraction. At the same time, its alpha properties constrict the peripheral vasculature, working together with the increased heart rate to increase perfusion. This would put less strain on the myocardium. Because of this, epinephrine may be better than Isuprel for treatment of complete heart block refractory to atropine (in the absence of an external pacemaker).

An epinephrine drip is mixed exactly the same way as an Isuprel drip. You take 1 milligram of epinephrine, mix it in a 250 cc bag of D_5W, and titrate it to the desired effect.

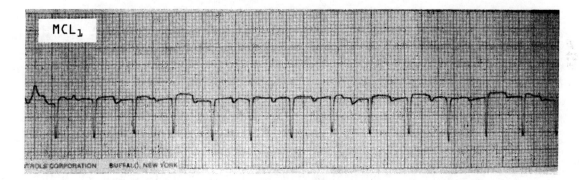

FIGURE 1.19

We didn't have an external pacemaker when we ran this call. So we hooked up an epinephrine drip and managed to increase this patient's heart rate to about 120 (Figure 1.19). His blood pressure came up to about 140 systolic, and his level of consciousness came up to actively combative. After the four-point restraints were in place, he received D_{50} and narcan, with little significant effect.

We got this patient into the emergency room, where a transcutaneous pacemaker was immediately hooked up. As they weaned him off the epinephrine drip, his heart rate proceeded to fall. But as soon as it got down to the right rate, the transcutaneous pacer kicked in. They tried for 6 hours to wean him off the pacer, but he stayed in complete heart block. They finally took him to the cath-lab and he received a permanent pacemaker.

The next day, in the coronary care unit, this patient admitted to smoking four rocks of crack cocaine just prior to the whole episode. Crack cocaine was the probable genesis of his cardiac problems.

TRANSIENT VENTRICULAR ASYSTOLE

The last in the reclassifications of A-V heart blocks is *transient ventricular asystole*. I have a little bit of concern with the way this classification was named because it's not always transient! Sometimes, it's *permanent* ventricular asystole.

There are primarily two causes of transient ventricular asystole; one is vagal stimulation, and the other is spontaneous occurrence. (There actually is a third type, the phase-4 phenomenon, but this phenomenon is mostly theoretical. The phase-4 phenomenon has to do with action potentials, which are discussed later in this text.)

Transient ventricular asystole is the failure (absence) of ventricular conduction despite the presence of atrial impulses. It is similar to complete heart block, except that it is associated with reluctant subsidiary pacemakers. This means that no impulses go through to the ventricles anymore—there is no A-V conduction and neither the junction nor the ventricles take over as pacemakers to fire the heart.

Rules for Transient Ventricular Asystole

Causes: (1) vagal stimulation and (2) spontaneous occurrence.

Failure (absence) of A-V conduction despite the presence of atrial impulses.

A reluctant subsidiary pacemaker (no junctional or ventricular QRS complexes).

As you may imagine, this can be a bad situation.

Our next patient was in a coronary care unit. He had an episode of wide-beat tachycardia that was converted with carotid sinus massage. Figure 1.20 is his EKG after the carotid sinus massage. Would you say that this was a successful conversion? At least he isn't in the wide-beat tachycardia anymore!

What would you call this rhythm? The atria are beating at a rate greater than 100 per minute. And there is a long period of time—26.5 seconds—where there is no subsidiary pacemaker generating ventricular complexes. So it's atrial tachycardia with ventricular asystole. I have to admire the intestinal fortitude of a coronary care unit staff that can wait 26.5 seconds for the next QRS complex.

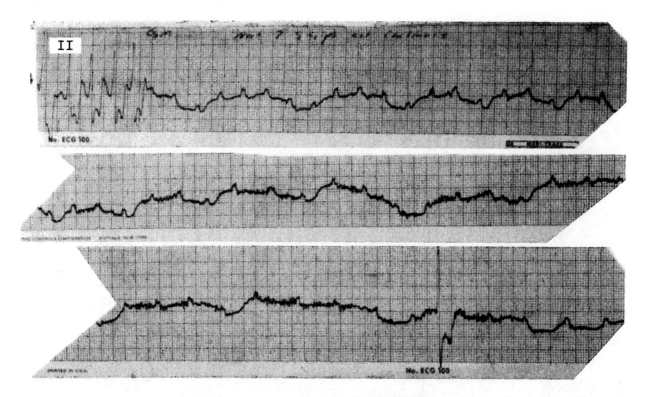

FIGURE 1.20

The rate slowly picked up (Figure 1.21) without intervention of any kind and managed to get up to a rate of about 76 with 2:1 conduction. This produced adequate perfusion, and this particular patient did fine.

Transient ventricular asystole is one of the things you have to worry about when you're converting wide-beat tachycardias by any means. If you work in an EMS system that does not allow carotid massage, it's probably because the person who wrote your protocols has had an experience like the one depicted in this case study. The transient ventricular asystole in Figures 1.20 and 1.21 was produced by the vagal stimulation of carotid sinus massage. This phenomenon was not widely recognized until after the advent of coronary care units in 1962.

The discovery of vagally induced transient ventricular asystole probably went something like this: A nurse was sitting at the nursing station, watching the unit's EKG monitors, when Mr. Jones in room 6 went into ventricular asystole. So the nurse hit the alarm button for a cardiac arrest. Everyone came running, lab coats flapping in the breeze behind them, pushing the crash cart to room 6. Upon their arrival, they found Mr. Jones perched on the bed pan trying to have a bowel movement. However, by this time, Mr. Jones's QRS complexes had returned. Transient ventricular asystole.

Perhaps you've had a few cardiac arrests where you find the patient in cardiac arrest between the commode and the tub. It's a reasonable possibility that the vagal stimulation of bearing down to have a bowel movement caused ventricular asystole—but unfortunately, it wasn't transient. This is the reason patients receive stool softeners in the CCU—so that they don't have to bear down too hard to have a BM.

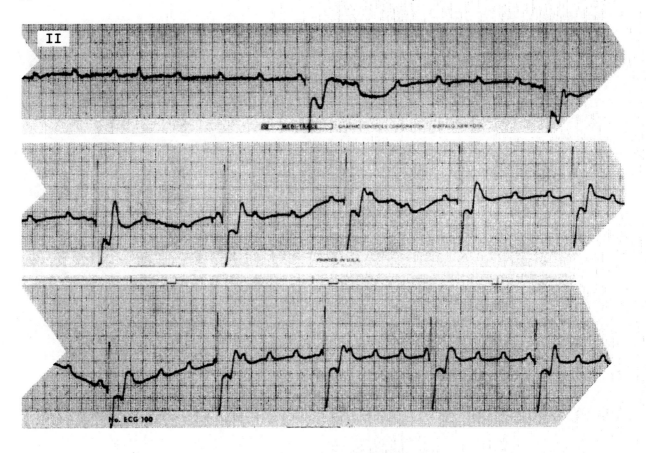

FIGURE 1.21

Spontaneous transient ventricular asystole is the type most likely to become *permanent* ventricular asystole. It is usually the fatal end stage of untreated type II A-V heart block. There are two key concepts here: fatal and type II. Spontaneous transient ventricular asystole is usually the fatal end stage of all type II blocks: occasional dropped beats type II, 2:1 block type II, or high-grade A-V block type II.

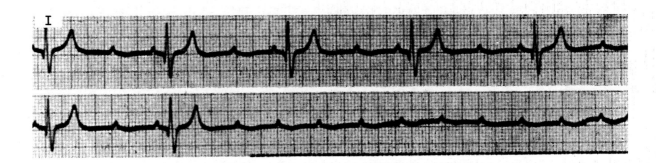

FIGURE 1.22 (Reproduced by permission of Dr. Henry J. L. Marriott, Director of Clinical Research and Education, Rogers Heart Foundation, St. Anthony's Hospital, St. Petersburg,

Remember this guy? Figure 1.22 is the EKG of the patient with cardiac syncope and high-grade A-V block type II that we looked at in Figure 1.14. He has nonconducted P waves hidden in each T wave, followed by another dropped P wave, with only every third P wave conducting to the ventricles (a 3:1 conduction ratio). What has happened to his rhythm in the lower strip of Figure 1.22? It became a sinus tachycardia with ventricular asystole.

What happened to this patient is that, initially, he had a permanent right bundle branch block, with an intermittent left bundle branch block. The first sinus impulse in the top strip conducted down the left bundle branch, creating a wide QRS complex. Then the sinus node fired again (hidden in the P wave), but the left bundle branch had become blocked. The sinus node fired again, and the left bundle branch was still blocked. The third sinus impulse found the left bundle branch conducting again. Then the cycle repeated. It continued to repeat until the bottom strip.

In the bottom strip, the left bundle branch block stopped being intermittent and became permanent. The seventh P wave of the bottom strip should have found the left bundle branch conducting again. But it was still blocked. The eighth sinus impulse was still blocked. The next one, still blocked. And it just stayed blocked.

At this point, if you had either a transcutaneous or an implantable pacemaker in place, you would flip the switch on. Hopefully, the pacemaker would capture and the heart would mechanically respond. Otherwise, this patient's prognosis would be rather grim.

SUMMARY

That's the reclassification of A-V blocks. The intent of this system of reclassified A-V blocks is to provide a plain English description of what's going on with the heart. It allows you to make safer, more appropriate treatment decisions for the customers you serve.

REFERENCES

1. Marriott, Henry J. L.: *Practical Electrocardiography*, 8th ed., 1988; Williams & Wilkins, Baltimore.
2. Kempe, K. Henry et al., "Battered Child." *JAMA* July 7, 1962; Vol. 181:17–24.

CHAPTER 2

Bundle Branch Blocks

I don't think there is such a thing as an "advanced" EKG class or an "advanced" EKG textbook. There are only EKGs and people who can read them with varying levels of expertise. If the emergency medical dispatcher has a patient on the telephone who sounds like he has a cardiac problem, how will she know whether to send a basic or an advanced EKG interpreter? If you hook up a patient and the monitor displays an "advanced EKG," but you've only had a "basic" class, do you call for an "advanced EKG" person? It doesn't work like that. Patients are at the mercy of whoever is caring for them, trusting the caregiver to read their EKG accurately regardless of its difficulty.

Some of you may have read the articles I've written in JEMS, titled "Cardiology Practicum." My co-author for those articles, Syd Canan, is also a co-author for this text. Syd has a favorite quote from cardiologist Gerald Gordon, M.D., that I certainly believe: "To know bundle branch blocks is to know cardiology."

When I teach a "basic" EKG class for people who have never before looked at an electrocardiogram, I quickly go through the anatomy and electrophysiology of the heart. Then I have everybody take EKGs of each other. I quickly talk about identifying P waves, QRS complexes, and T waves; how to measure the different waves; and how to assess the rates. And the next thing I teach is bundle branch blocks. Right off the bat. Because if you have a good understanding of bundle branch blocks, it makes understanding the rest of EKG interpretation much easier.

It is important when diagnosing bundle branch blocks to look at more than one lead. Actually, this is important when diagnosing most things in electrocardiography. In order to make a good diagnosis, assessing a single lead is seldom enough.

When you drive along a street, has the back of a person walking along the sidewalk ever caught your attention? The person strikes you as being rather attractive, so you slow down as you drive by. Once you are past the person, you look over your shoulder, and, "Oooh, that person was not as attractive as I originally thought!" Initially, you looked at that pedestrian from only one point of view—and made a "misdiagnosis." But as soon as you looked from a different view, you had a more complete picture. Your "diagnosis" was affected by it. You drove away!

In Figure 2.1, how wide is the QRS in lead I? About 0.08 seconds. How wide is the QRS in lead II? It's 0.12 seconds. How about in lead III? 0.12 seconds also. Guess what? This is a simultaneous tracing. You're seeing the same beat simultaneously—from three points of view. How can the QRS in lead I be shorter than the QRS in leads II and III? It can't. Some leads simply show a clearer beginning and end to the QRS complex.

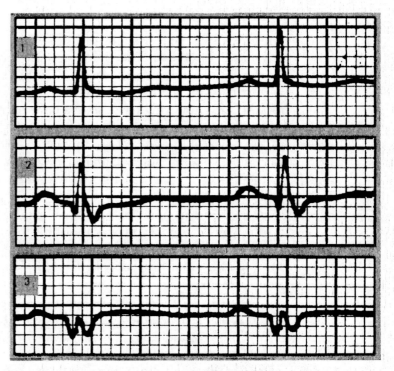

FIGURE 2.1 (Henry J. L. Marriott, *Practical Electrocardiography*, 8th ed., 1988; Williams & Wilkins, Baltimore.)

In order to determine the width of a QRS complex, you need to assess more than one lead so that you can find the one with the widest complex and the clearest beginning and end. That will be the true width of the patient's QRS complex.

Figure 2.2 provides markers for the beginning and end of the QRS complexes from Figure 2.1. Look at the markers for lead II. You can clearly see the beginning and end of that QRS. It clearly measures 0.12 seconds. Lead I is exactly the same QRS complex shown in lead II, but it simply isn't quite as clear in that particular lead. The last part of it blends into the base line and creates the illusion of a narrow QRS complex. This is why several leads, or views, of any electrocardiogram are essential. Different views provide a more complete picture.

The same thing happens with the premature atrial complexes (PACs) that some people call "funny-looking beats" (FLBs). They may well be premature *ventricular* complexes (PVCs). If you truly want to know which they are, look at them in more than one lead.

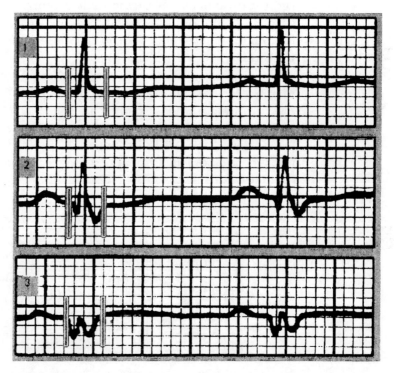

FIGURE 2.2 (Henry J. L. Marriott, *Practical Electrocardiography*, 8th ed., 1988; Williams & Wilkins, Baltimore.)

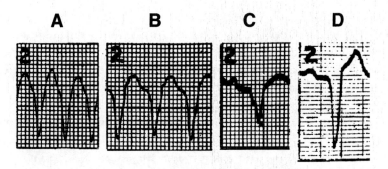

FIGURE 2.3 (Henry J. L. Marriott, *Practical Electrocardiography*, 8th ed., 1988; Williams & Wilkins, Baltimore.)

Okay. Look at Figure 2.3 and forget about the P waves. For those of you accustomed to monitoring patients in lead II, is the QRS complex in strip A ventricular or supraventricular? If it's supraventricular, is it a right bundle branch block or a left bundle branch block? If it's ventricular, is it right ventricular tachycardia or left ventricular tachycardia? How about strip B? Is this right ventricular tachycardia, left ventricular tachycardia, left bundle branch block, or right bundle branch block? What about strip C? And D?

Think about the purpose of EKG monitoring. The primary reason is to watch for changes. People who monitor patient rhythms solely in lead II have a problem when a patient in a perfectly "normal sinus rhythm" goes into something like what you see in strip A in Figure 2.3. All they can say is, "Ooh, the patient's EKG changed! I don't know what it is. I don't know what to do about it. Don't know how dangerous it is. But there's been a change!"

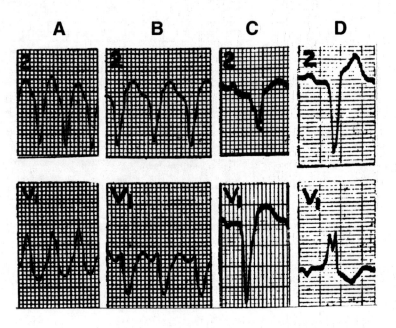

FIGURE 2.4 (Henry J. L. Marriott, *Practical Electrocardiography*, 8th ed., 1988; Williams & Wilkins, Baltimore).

On the other hand, people who monitor patient EKGs in MCL$_1$ have a much better chance of knowing what the change is and what to do about it. Figure 2.4 shows the MCL$_1$ tracing of the same complexes shown in Figure 2.3. By using the MCL$_1$ lead, I can tell you that strip A is a left ventricular tachycardia, strip B is a right ventricular tachycardia, strip C is a left bundle branch block, and strip D is a right bundle branch block.

Once you've recognized the true identities of these rhythms, you'll know that strips A and B should be treated by following your ventricular tachycardia protocol. And strips C and D, should be treated by following your supraventricular tachycardia protocol. Using the wrong protocol or medications to treat either set of patients could cause them serious—even fatal—complications.

Why would anyone monitor a patient in lead II when it provides such dangerously limited information? I encourage people to monitor patients in a lead that will not only allow them to know "something's happened!," but to know what has happened. Knowing what has happened gives you an idea of what to do about it.

The best lead for monitoring patient EKGs is MCL$_1$. That stands for *modified chest left*, not modified chest "lead" or "Marriott's chest lead—although both are common misunderstandings. Modified chest left is an adaptation of the old "chest left" lead, which connected the chest and left arm. It's virtually the same lead as V$_1$ of a 12-lead electrocardiogram.

Differential diagnosis of right or left bundle branch blocks, right or left ventricular tachycardias, and right or left ventricular ectopy is easier when you use MCL$_1$. And you don't want to try this in lead II. It won't work.

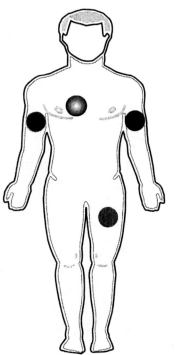

To Run MCL 1

- Leave the Lead Selector on III

- Move the Red Cable to the 4th ICS just to the Right of the Sternum

Lead placement for MCL$_1$ includes placing the negative electrode on the left arm and a positive electrode in the fourth intercostal space just to the right of the sternum. Not on the fifth rib. Not at the right nipple line. Not at all the other places people place it. But at the fourth intercostal space, just to the right of the sternum.

If you have a hard time finding the fourth intercostal space, try this. Gently find the suprasternal notch, and slide your finger down to the dip and bump in the middle of the sternum. That's where the manubrium and the gladiolus bones join (also known as the angle of Louis). Slide your finger to the right side of the sternum onto the rib cage. You'll be at the second intercostal space, which is between the second and third ribs. Go down to the next interspace (third intercostal space), then the next, and you've found the fourth intercostal space. The positive electrode goes *right* next to the sternum.

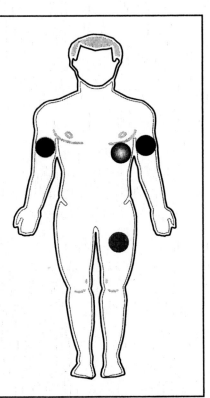

To Run MCL 6

- Leave the Lead Selector on III

- Locate the 5th ICS at the left Mid-Clavicular Line
- Place the Electrode at the left Mid-Axillary Line horizontal to this point
- Move the Red Cable to this Electrode

Another lead you'll need to be familiar with when we get into differential diagnosis of supraventricular versus ventricular tachycardia is MCL$_6$. Proper placement of both the MCL$_1$ and MCL$_6$ electrodes is essential to the differential diagnosis of supraventricular and ventricular tachycardia.

To place MCL$_6$, leave the negative electrode on the left arm. Place the positive lead of MCL$_6$ on the left midaxillary line. After placing the positive electrode for MCL$_1$, slide your finger across the sternum to the patient's left chest, still in the fourth intercostal space. Slide down over one more rib to find the fifth intercostal space. From there, draw a line around into the left midaxillary line (underneath the arm pit). That's where the electrode goes for MCL_6. Do not follow the intercostal space or rib. The electrode should be placed in the left midaxillary line at the *level* where the fifth intercostal space joins the sternum.

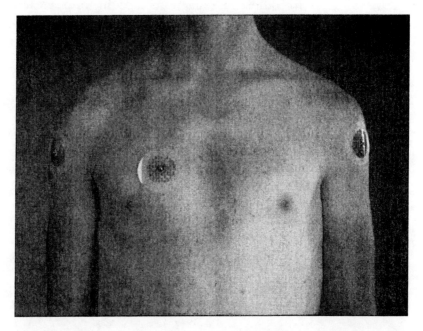

PHOTO 2:1 MCL_1 lead placement. (Michal Heron Photography.)

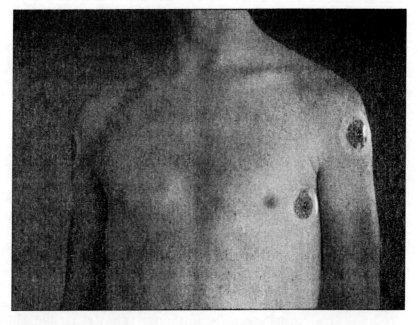

PHOTO 2:2 MCL_6 lead placement. (Michal Heron Photography.)

ANATOMY AND PHYSIOLOGY (A&P) REVIEW

In our workshops, we invite participants to sit back and relax through the A&P portion of the bundle branch block discussion. This is because at the end of this next section we provide a simple and easy to remember strategy for differential diagnosis of right from left bundle branch block. In fact, if you are one of those people who likes to skip to the "quick fix," easy strategy, you are welcome to turn to page 55 and dive right into stuff you can use!

By any chance, did you ever happen to see the movie, *Texas Chain Saw Massacre*? A scene in that movie showed a guy getting cut in half, horizontally, across the middle of his chest. Well, that's how the anatomic view of the heart in these next few figures is obtained.

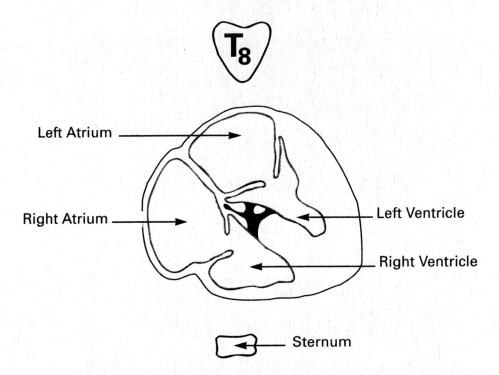

FIGURE 2.5 Horizontal cross section of the heart, viewed from a superior point of view.

In Figure 2.5 you can see that the sternum is in front, and (approximately) the eighth thoracic vertebrae is in back. This view shows us the right atrium, left atrium, right ventricle, left ventricle, and the interventricular septum.

Unfortunately, our anatomic textbooks and anatomy classes have misled us a little bit. Let's say that after reading this text, you became extremely angry with me. You foster this anger until you happen to meet me at an EMS conference. There you stabbed me with a knife in the fourth intercostal space just to the left of my sternum. What would be the first cardiac structure the knife would touch after it pierced my pericardium? That structure would be my *right* ventricle.

Now, does it make any sense at all that you can put a knife into the *left* side of somebody's chest, and hit a structure that has the term "right" attached to it? And is the *right* ventricle really to the *right* of the left ventricle? Not much. It's more *in front of* the left ventricle. Realistically, they should be called the anterior ventricle and the posterior ventricle, because, anatomically, that's the way they sit. But I've already rocked a few boats with this text. I can't change all the anatomical terms so soon after promoting the reclassification of first-, second-, and third-degree heart blocks! However, it's important for you to understand that the terms right and left don't correlate with the anatomical position of the ventricles. In order to be able to diagnose bundle branch blocks, you need to understand that the right ventricle is anterior to the left ventricle.

Also, when my right atrium is full of blood and it contracts, in which direction does the blood squirt? Most of the time, textbooks picture the heart as this dangley thing with the atria above the ventricles. Naturally, we would imagine the blood being squirted down from the atria to the ventricle. Well, it doesn't squirt down, it moves across. The atria are more to the "side" of the ventricles than "above" them.

Normal electrical activation of the heart occurs in the following manner: The sinus node fires and the impulse travels the internodal pathways to the A-V node. From the A-V node the impulse travels to the bundle of His, which is only about a centimeter long. Then it divides into the left and right bundle branches.

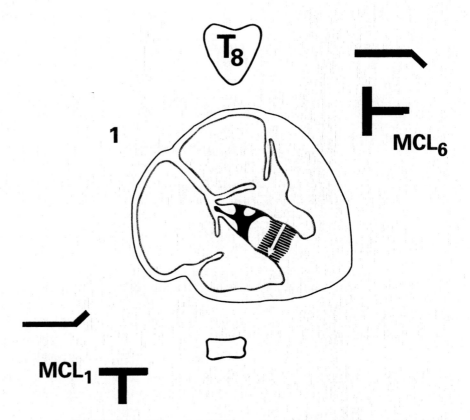

FIGURE 2.6 Normal, initial septal activation of the ventricles.

Normal activation of the ventricles is first started by some fibers that come off of the left bundle branch (see Figure 2.6). These fibers are located in the wall of the left side of the septum in the left septal endocardium. The first activation of the ventricles is that of the impulse firing across the interventricular septum, from the left to the right.

That impulse travels toward the positive electrode of MCL_1, which you have (properly) placed in the fourth intercostal space just to the right of the sternum. This is what creates the small, upright r wave, the first deflection of a normal QRS complex in MCL_1.

In MCL_6, the impulse is traveling away from the positive electrode, creating a small, negative q wave as the first deflection of a normal QRS complex there.

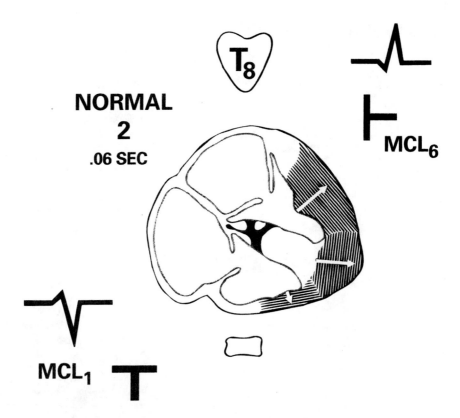

FIGURE 2.7 Normal completion of ventricular activation.

Next, both ventricles fire simultaneously (Figure 2.7). The left may fire just a bit before the right, but for all practical purposes, when you're reading the electrocardiogram, they basically fire simultaneously *in a normal heart.*

The electrocardiogram can only pick up impulses that are "left over"—impulses that aren't canceled out by opposing impulses. According to Dr. Marriott, it actually picks up only about 10 percent of the total impulses generated within the heart. The left ventricle contains 75 percent of the mass of the heart. It is composed of much more muscle mass than the right ventricle; it is about six times thicker. Consequently, an impulse traveling through the left ventricle will contribute more to the QRS complex than the impulse traveling through the smaller, thinner right ventricular wall. Thus, the majority of what you see on the electrocardiogram is contributed by the left ventricle.

So in MCL$_1$, after the initial small r wave comes a deep left ventricular-generated S wave (Figure 2.7). The majority of forces have traveled away from the positive electrode in MCL$_1$, creating a primarily negative complex.

In MCL$_6$, the majority of forces are traveling toward the positive electrode, creating an upright complex. After the initial q wave comes a tall R wave.

The normal amount of time required to activate the septum and the ventricles is about 0.06 seconds. A QRS width of less than 0.12 seconds is considered to have normal duration.

RIGHT BUNDLE BRANCH BLOCK

If a patient has a disease process that blocks the right bundle branch, the initial impulse of the ventricles is not going to be changed at all. This is because initial ventricular activation is from the left endocardium through to the right. The first part of the QRS complex will be identical to a normal complex (Figure 2.6): a small r wave in MCL_1 and a small q wave in MCL_6. This is important to remember when differentiating between a *supraventricular* rhythm and a *ventricular* tachycardia.

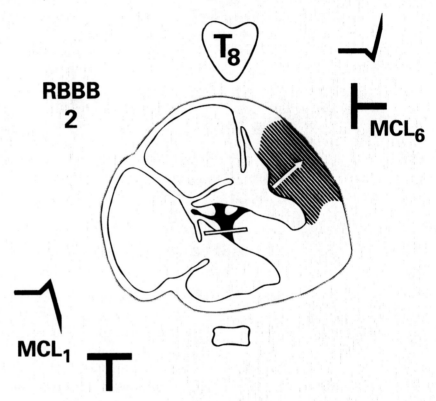

FIGURE 2.8 Ventricular activation (*after* normal septal activation) in the presence of a right bundle branch block.

Next, the left ventricle fires all by itself, since the right bundle branch is blocked (Figure 2.8). That still follows normal QRS patterns. What we're used to seeing on a normal electrocardiogram is primarily the left ventricle firing. So that results in an S wave in MCL_1 and an R wave in MCL_6.

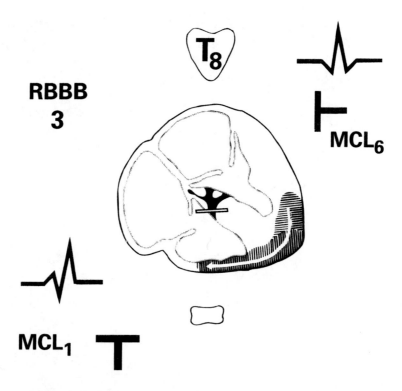

FIGURE 2.9 Late right ventricular activation in the presence of a right bundle branch block.

The right ventricle is still going to be stimulated, but it gets activated via a different route because of the blocked bundle branch (Figure 2.9). Activation goes through the muscular wall instead of through the electrical conduction system. The impulse has to cross over the interventricular septum and then fire the right ventricle via the muscle. This is much slower than having the impulse travel through the His–Purkinje system (which is blocked). What we have now is a right ventricle that is firing *after* the left ventricle. Since it is firing unopposed, the electrocardiogram inscribes its impulses. In MCL_1, these impulses are traveling toward the positive electrode, causing a positive deflection. And they are going away from the positive electrode in MCL_6, causing a negative deflection there.

Often you will hear this MCL$_1$ pattern described as "R-S-R prime" (RSR'). It is the classic right bundle branch block pattern and should *only* be looked for in MCL$_1$. Seeing this pattern in any other lead, especially lead II, means nothing. Figure 2.10 is an MCL$_1$ EKG and shows an example of RSR' right bundle branch block pattern.

A bundle branch block creates a wider QRS complex. Normally, it takes about 0.06 seconds to fire the ventricles. With a bundle branch block it takes about another 0.06 seconds. This creates a QRS complex that is 0.12 seconds wide or wider.

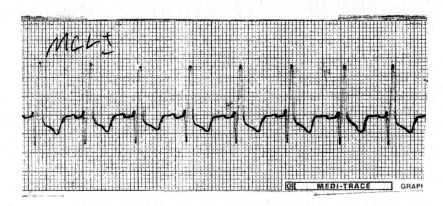

FIGURE 2.10 Classic right bundle branch block pattern ("R-S-R prime" - RSR') in MCL$_1$.

I'd also like you to notice what portion of the QRS complex in Figure 2.10 is inscribed by the ventricle that is blocked. Because the right bundle branch is blocked, the right ventricle is the last to fire. Whichever ventricle has the blocked bundle branch produces the very last part of the QRS complex. Therefore, the last part of the QRS complex is what we look at for differential diagnosis of bundle branch blocks.

LEFT BUNDLE BRANCH BLOCK

If the patient has a left bundle branch block, the initial firing of the ventricle will be altered. This is because the interventricular septum normally fires from the left endocardium through to the right.

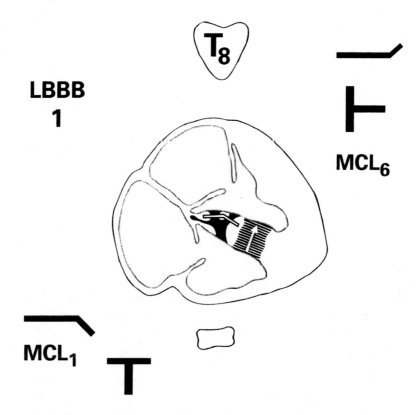

FIGURE 2.11 Altered initial septal activation in the presence of approximately 70 percent of left bundle branch blocks.

In the majority of hearts with left bundle branch block, the initial impulse travels from the right endocardium to the left (activated by some septal fibers off the right bundle branch) (Figure 2.11). Now the initial impulse is going *away from* the positive electrode in MCL_1, so we see a small q wave in MCL_1, instead of an r wave. In MCL_6, the initial impulse is going *toward* the positive electrode, producing an r wave instead of the normal q wave.

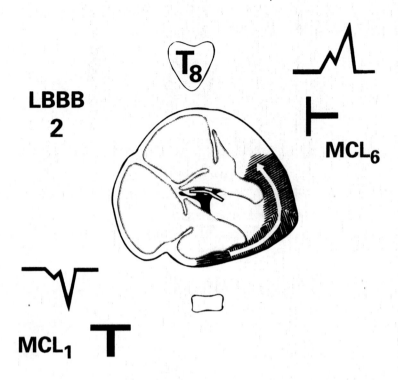

FIGURE 2.12 Unopposed right ventricular activation followed by late left ventricular activation, in the presence of a left bundle branch block.

The next thing that happens is that the right ventricle fires unopposed. That is, the left ventricle isn't doing anything yet. This may produce a small r wave in MCL_1 and sometimes a small s wave in MCL_6. Then, after the right ventricle fires, the impulse travels across the interventricular septum and fires the left ventricle (Figure 2.12). The impulse is traveling away from the positive electrode in MCL_1, producing a deep, fat S wave, and toward the positive electrode in MCL_6, producing a tall, fat R wave. This altered route takes longer. It takes 0.12 seconds or longer to finally activate the left ventricle.

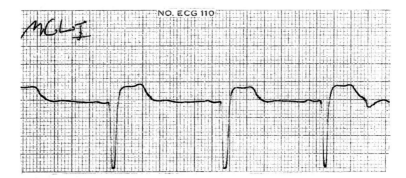

FIGURE 2.13 Approximately 70 percent of left bundle branch blocks will show this pattern in MCL_1 (no initial r wave).

And again, as you can see in Figure 2.13, the terminal portion of the QRS complex shows left ventricular activation since that's the bundle branch that is blocked.

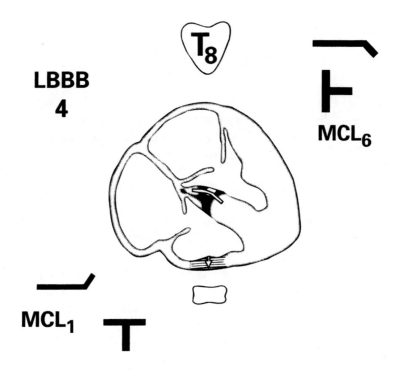

FIGURE 2.14 Approximately 30 percent of left bundle branch blocks have initial right ventricular activation, creating small, initial r wave.

In a small percentage of patients with left bundle branch block, the very first thing to be activated is the free wall of the right ventricle (Figure 2.14). Either the fibers of the right bundle branch are not tied into the septum, or there is a different conduction velocity (speed of conduction) within the Purkinje fibers. This means that the right ventricle gets activated before the septum or left ventricle.

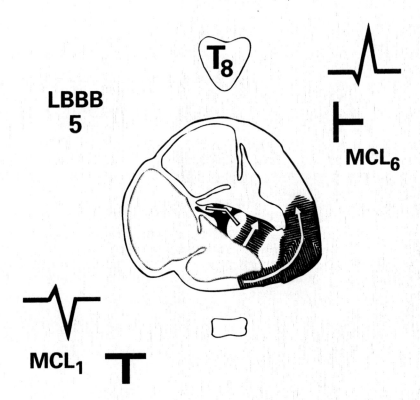

FIGURE 2.15 Completion of right ventricular activation followed by late left ventricular activation in the presence of a left bundle branch block.

When the right ventricle is activated first, in MCL_1 it inscribes a very small, thin r wave for the initial deflection. It is important to know the difference between a thin r wave and a fat R wave in MCL_1. Later in this text, I'll share the reason with you. In MCL_6, the initial deflection will be a small, thin q wave.

After right ventricular depolarization, the impulse travels across the septum (Figure 2.15) to activate the left ventricle. This writes a deep S wave in MCL_1 and a tall R wave in MCL_6 and produces a QRS complex that is 0.12 seconds wide or wider.

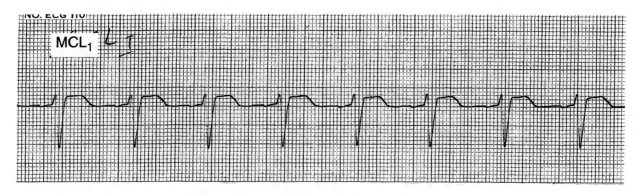

FIGURE 2.16 Approximately 30 percent of left bundle branch blocks will show this pattern in MCL$_1$ (having a small, initial r wave).

Please note that in MCL$_1$ of Figure 2.16 the terminal portion of the QRS complex is negative in 100 percent of the left bundle branch blocks. Why do I keep mentioning that? I'll tell you now:

Years ago, I was in a hotel meeting room in Boulder, Colorado, teaching an EMT-Intermediate class. One student, Willard Crary, and I were engaged in the ongoing struggle of trying to find the simplest way to differentiate left from right bundle branch blocks. Suddenly, Willard said, "Well, hey! This is just like driving a car!" And it turns out that he was correct. When you drive your automobile, do you use your turn signal? If you do, you can effortlessly differentially diagnose left from right bundle branch blocks. Here's the way you do it:

Step 1. Find the J point of a QRS complex in MCL$_1$. The J point is the end of the QRS complex, the *junction* between the end of the QRS complex and the beginning of the S-T segment.

> The J point is the junction of the end of the QRS complex and the beginning of the S-T segment.

Step 2. Place your pen on the J-point (Photo 2.4) and draw a horizontal line back into the QRS complex. This creates a triangle.

Step 3. Fill in the triangle, and you have a bundle branch block indicator (Figure 2.17).

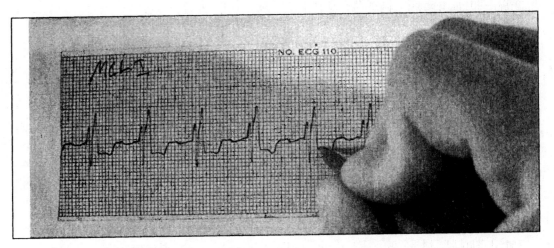

PHOTO 2.3 Place your pen on the J-point and draw a horizontal line back into the QRS complex, creating a triangle, then color it in.

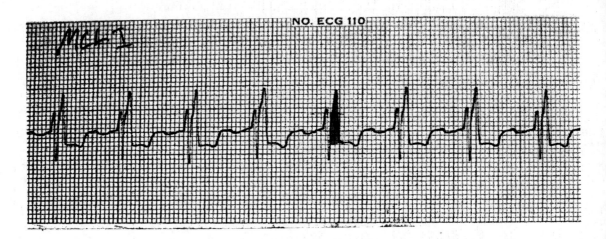

FIGURE 2.17 The colored-in triangle is a bundle branch block indicator that corresponds with the turn signal indicator of a car. When the QRS complex is greater than 0.12 seconds long, a triangle pointing up is a right bundle branch block, a triangle pointing sown is a left bundle branch block.

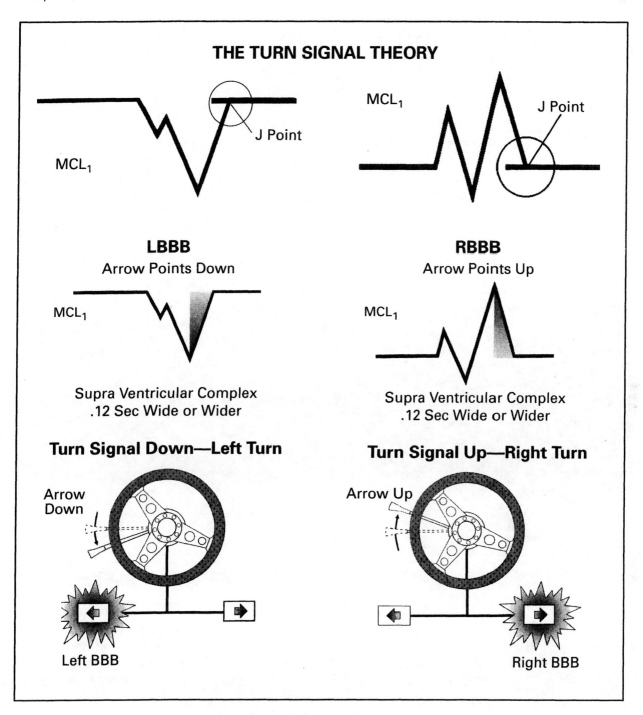

This is called the *turn signal theory* because you push the turn signal
lever *up* to signal a right turn and *down* to signal a left turn. As you can see
looking at the Turn Signal Theory box, if the triangle points up, you have
a right bundle branch block. If the triangle points down, you have a left
bundle branch block. Remember, this technique *only* applies to supraventricular QRS complexes that are 0.12 seconds wide or wider and can *only*
be performed in MCL_1.

At this point, someone usually always asks me, "How can you tell where the J point is if the QRS complexes in MCL$_1$ aren't clear?"

Remember Figures 2.1 and 2.2? You have to look at different leads. Make it a habit to run leads I, II, III, and MCL$_1$. Find the widest QRS complex with the clearest beginning and end. Then make your QRS measurement. If the clearest QRS complex is in a lead other than MCL$_1$, take that measurement and transfer it to the QRS complexes in MCL$_1$. Then you can find the "hidden" J point in MCL$_1$ and draw your arrow.

Personally, I love coloring. But, if you get tired of drawing and coloring in triangles, you will start to visualize them. Then you'll discover that, when the final deflection of a wide supraventricular QRS complex in MCL$_1$ is positive, it is a right bundle branch block. And when the final deflection of a wide supraventricular QRS complex in MCL$_1$ is negative, it is a left bundle branch block.

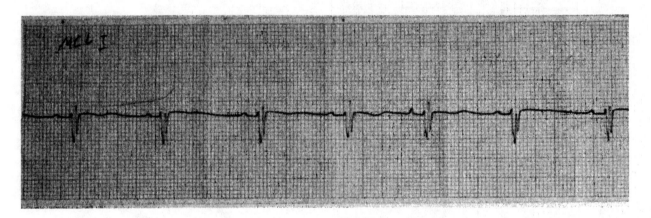

FIGURE 2.18

Let's practice with the EKG strip in Figure 2.18. Find the J point, draw in your arrow, and what do you have? The arrow points down, so you have a left bundle branch block, right?

No! Trick strip. The QRS complexes are only 0.10 seconds wide. This strip does not include a bundle branch block. This is a 15-year-old male's EKG strip and is an example of a normal juvenile pattern. In order to diagnose a bundle branch block, remember that you must first have a QRS complex of 0.12 seconds wide or wider. (Some texts say that 0.11 seconds is wide enough for a right bundle branch block. Your choice.) The important thing is to remember that a bizarre QRS complex does not a bundle branch block make, unless it is 0.12 seconds wide or wider. And also remember, this won't work in lead II.

Okay. Let's really practice now.

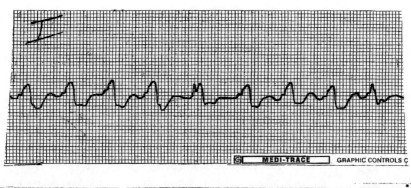

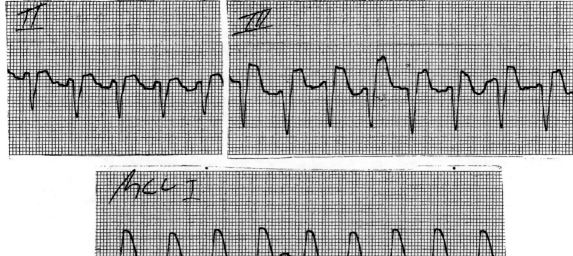

FIGURE 2.19

In Figure 2.19 you see leads I, II, III, and MCL$_1$. First, you should notice that the QRS complexes are wide. There are P waves in front of each QRS complex, so it looks like this patient has a sinus tachycardia. Now look at MCL$_1$ to evaluate whether the patient has a left or a right bundle branch block. On this strip, some people have a hard time determining where the J point is in MCL$_1$. Look at lead II and measure the width of the QRS complex. In this case, the QRS is very wide (0.16 seconds). Once you have your 0.16-second measurement, go to the MCL$_1$ lead's QRS. It's pretty clear where the beginning of the QRS complex is. Measure 0.16 seconds from there, and make a mark there for the J point. Draw a line back in toward the center of the QRS complex and fill in the triangle. You will have a triangle that is pointing downward. When you push the turn signal downward to make a turn in your car, you are going to make a left turn. Thus, in this case, you have a left bundle branch block.

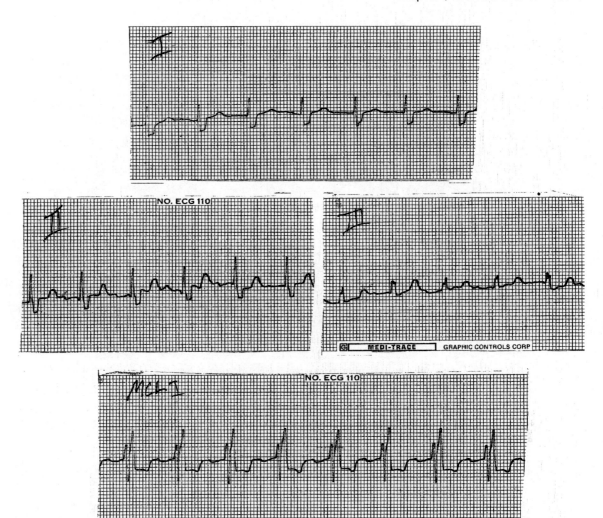

FIGURE 2.20

This patient (Figure 2.20) has a sinus rhythm at a rate just under 100 with a wide QRS complex. Go to the MCL₁ lead. In this case it's easy to clearly identify the end of the QRS complex, or the J point. Put your pen there, and draw a line back into the center of the QRS complex. As soon as you've touched another line, fill in the little triangle that's created. The little triangle points up. This patient has a right bundle branch block.

SUMMARY

At the end of this section in our workshops, we ask participants to raise their hands if they knew how to diagnose bundle branch blocks when they walked into the room at the beginning of the day. Usually, only one or two hands go up. Then we ask the question, "Well, how many of you know how to identify right from left bundle branch blocks now?" Sometimes it takes a second or two, but before long all the hands in the room come up. That's when we smile broadly and ask, "Is that worth the price of admission, or what?"

CHAPTER 3

Determining
the Electrical Axis

Determining the electrical axis of the heart is one of those things we've traditionally been told that "paramedics don't need to know." Once again defying old beliefs, let us disregard this erroneous tradition and learn how to determine the electrical axis of the heart. In this book we will help you understand precisely why paramedics *do* need to know how to do this.

Axis can be defined as the general direction of electrical impulses as they travel through the heart.

There are several usable methods for determining axis. First, there is the hexaxial reference system. You take lines representing the three sides of Einthoven's triangle (the three limb leads) and cross them over each other. Then you take lines representing aVR, aVL, and aVF, crossing those together with the others. This creates a wheel of six bisecting lines, to which you add degrees and pluses and minuses. Then you find the tallest QRS complex of the limb leads and then the one that has the most isoelectric complex. You plot them out on this wheel, performing incredible mathematical acrobatics, and end up determining the axis.

Or you can use Dr. M. J. Goldman's method, as found in his text *Principles of Clinical Electrocardiography.*[1] This is where you determine the algebraic sum of the R and the S in lead I, and plot this value on the lead I axis of Goldman's diagram. Then you determine the algebraic sum of the R and the S in lead III to plot on lead III's axis of the diagram, and so on, and so forth, continuing through a five-step algebraic process to determine the axis.

You could learn either of these methods in less than an hour. After a few hours of practice, you could use either method to figure any EKG's axis accurately and consistently. But about six weeks from now, at three o'clock in the morning when you're in a stranger's living room, you'll rub the sleep out of your eyes, look at the person's EKG, and think "Axis? How did that go again?"

Obviously, I see little benefit in spending a lot of time and energy on these particular styles of learning axis. Instead, I came up with a quick, easy to use method of axis determination.

First, I looked at the axis of over a thousand 12-lead electrocardiograms, using both the hexaxial reference system and Goldman's system. Using this information, I developed a system to simplify the process. Unless you're reading fifteen or twenty 12-leads a day, I think you'll find this approach easier.

The first thing to do is get the lead placement right. Where do you put the electrodes on a patient when you're going to take an electrocardiogram? Have you ever looked at how the leads are labeled? The white one has an RA on it. That stands for *right arm*. The black lead is labeled LA. That stands for *left arm*. And the red lead is labeled LL, meaning *left leg*. So why are leads commonly placed on the chest and belly by emergency medical personnel both in and out of the hospital?

My guess is that it went something like this: When they first started coronary care units—in Kansas on May 20, 1962—they were very excited about being able to monitor multiple patients at a central nursing station. Initially, they hooked up the leads just like they always had. They used those attractive rubber wrist and ankle straps for the limb leads. But they soon discovered a problem with this. Every time a patient went to scratch an itch, or eat a bite of food, or (heaven forbid!) brush his teeth, it would look to the monitoring nurse as if Mr. Jones had just gone into ventricular fibrillation. So she would sound the alarm. As you can imagine, they rapidly tired of responding to false alarms. To minimize the miscellaneous artifact created by patient movement, they gradually moved the electrodes in to the chest and stomach.

For those of you who have done clinical time in coronary care units, what's one of the first things they do when somebody throws an arrhythmia? They call for a 12-lead electrocardiogram. They put the electrodes on the limbs (where they're supposed to be) and run a *diagnostic* 12-lead. Why do they do this? Because a diagnostic EKG requires more than just one lead, and it requires *correct lead placement*.

The right arm lead has to be on the right arm, the left arm lead on the left arm, and the left leg lead on the left leg. The biceps area is a good placement for the arm electrodes. The left leg electrode can go on the thigh or ankle, adjusted as necessary to accommodate the patient's clothing.

The chest is *not* the correct placement of electrodes for leads I, II, or III, (Figure 3.1). The stomach is also incorrect. And we've already discussed the importance of proper placement of the positive electrode in MCL_1 and MCL_6.

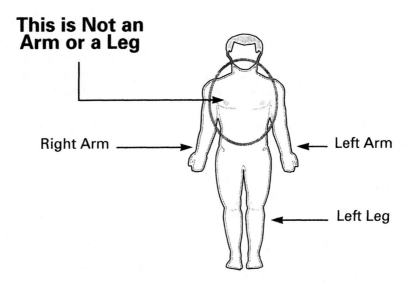

**This is Not an
Arm or a Leg**

Right Arm

Left Arm

Left Leg

FIGURE 3.1 The chest is *not* the correct placement of electrodes for leads I, II, or III.

Once you have recorded leads I, II, and III, you can determine the electrical axis. While you can determine the axis of P waves and T waves, the QRS axis contains the most useful information. Normally, the impulses start from the sinus node, which is basically in the upper right side of the body. Then the impulses travel downward, toward the ventricles—or the lower left side of the body. Normally conducted impulses travel toward the positive electrode in leads I, II, and III. Whenever an impulse travels toward a positive electrode, it inscribes an *upright* deflection. Therefore, an impulse traveling normal routes through the heart will inscribe a complex that is upright in lead I, lead II, and lead III (Figure 3.2).

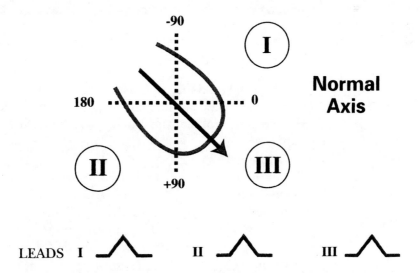

-90

I

180 0

**Normal
Axis**

II

III

+90

LEADS   I   II   III

FIGURE 3.2 The most normal electrical axis produces primarily upright (positive) complexes in leads I, II, and III.

If you have difficulty deciding whether a complex is more positive (upright) or more negative (downward), there are two different methods to use. You can count the number of millimeters the complex inscribes above the baseline and the number it inscribes below. Compare the two and determine which direction travels across the greater number of millimeters. That would be the primary direction of deflection.

Or you can use what I've heard called "the Jack Daniels cup" method. That's when you draw a line connecting the baseline of each end of the complex. If you filled each deflection away from the line with Jack Daniels, whichever one would hold more alcohol is the primary direction of deflection.

Sometimes, however, the amounts of deflection above and below the baseline are equivalent. This deflection is called *isoelectric*. An example of an isoelectric QRS complex would be the middle QRS complex in Figure 3.3. Look at Figure 3.3 and practice determining the primary direction of deflection with either of these two methods.

Is it Positive or Negative?

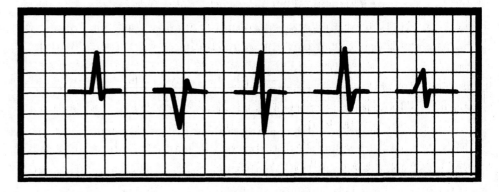

FIGURE 3.3

"Normal" axis is the easy one. Not only is it simple to identify, it makes sense. The "abnormal" axes (ak´sez; plural of axis) tend to sound confusing in explanation, but are easily identified on the electrocardiogram.

If the axis rotates upward, toward the patient's left, it is called a left axis deviation. Some left axis deviations are still considered normal. On the electrocardiogram, normal, or *physiologic*, left axis deviations—physiology being the study of what normally happens within the body—are recognized by an upright complex in lead I, either an upright or isoelectric complex in lead II, and a negative complex in lead III (Figure 3.4).

If the axis rotates further upward (left), it is called a *pathologic* left axis deviation—pathology being the study of disease processes. In a pathologic left axis deviation, you'll see an upright QRS complex in lead I and negative QRS complexes in leads II and III (Figure 3.5).

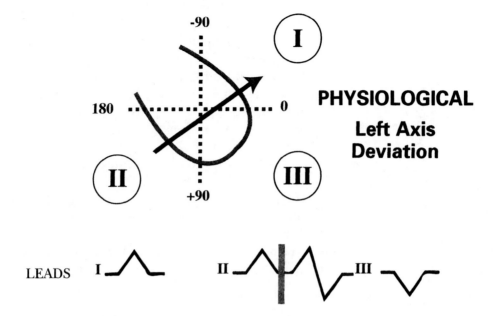

FIGURE 3.4 Some axes normally have a bit of a left axis deviation. An axis that is just a little bit left is called a physiologic left axis deviation. Physiologic left axis deviation produces complexes that are primarily upright (positive) in lead I and primarily downward (negative) complexes in lead III. Lead II may be either upright or isoelectric.

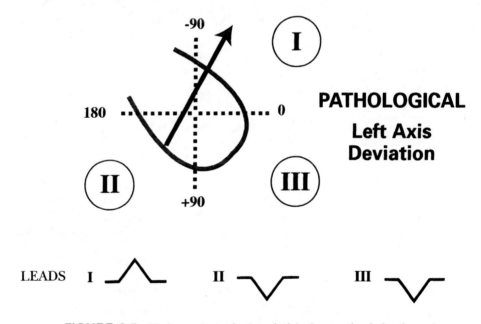

FIGURE 3.5 If the axis is deviated this far to the left, there is something wrong with the heart. Because pathology is the study of disease processes, an abnormal left axis deviation is called a pathologic left axis deviation. Pathologic left axis deviation produces complexes that are primarily upright (positive) in lead I and primarily downward (negative) complexes in both leads II and III.

All left axis deviations will have primarily upright (positive) complexes in lead I and primarily downward (negative) complexes in lead III. By looking at lead II, it's easy to differentiate physiologic from pathologic left axis deviation. If lead II is upright or isoelectric, the axis is physiologic and within normal limits. If lead II is negative, the axis is pathological left axis deviation, and thus part of a disease process.

Since there are normal and abnormal left axis deviations, you need to differentiate between the two in your diagnosis, verbal report, and written report. The importance of this differentiation will be made clear when we discuss hemiblocks.

If the axis deviates to the right, the impulse is now traveling away from the positive electrode in lead I and toward the positive electrode in lead III. This creates a negative or downward complex in lead I and a positive or upward complex in lead III. Lead II may be positive, isoelectric, or negative (Figure 3.6)

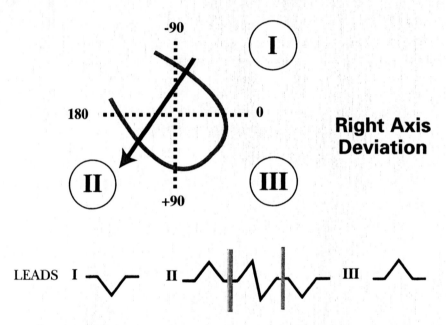

FIGURE 3.6 An electrical axis that travels away from the positive electrode in lead I (downward deflection) and ends up traveling toward the positive electrode in lead III (upright deflection) is considered a right axis deviation. Lead II can be positive, isoelectric, or negative. *All* right axis deviations are considered pathological.

Right axis deviations are not differentiated into physiological or pathological deviations. Right axis deviations are all considered to be pathological.

What would the heart's axis be if all the complexes were negative—negative in leads I, II, and III? Exactly the opposite of "normal." We call this situation a *right shoulder axis*. Some authors call it "extreme left," "extreme right," or "No Man's Land." I've found that, since it points to the right shoulder, the term *right shoulder axis* is easiest to describe and remember. This particular type of axis is associated with ventricular dysrhythmias, which start at the opposite end of the heart from the normally occurring sinus impulses (Figure 3.7).

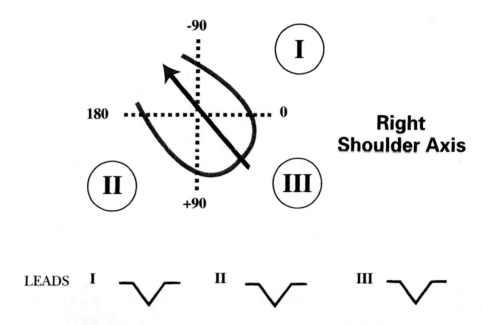

FIGURE 3.7 Right shoulder axis is associated with ventricular dysrhythmias. Negative deflections in leads I, II, and III indicate a right shoulder axis.

One reason you should always run leads I, II, and III on somebody with a wide complex tachycardia is this: if the complexes are negative in all these leads, the rhythm is more likely to be ventricular than supraventricular.

Now, I'm a little bit reluctant to show you this last axis. Originally, I put together a system of five axis patterns: normal, physiologic left, pathologic left, right axis, and right shoulder axis. I taught my system with the message that "if you know these five patterns, you can quickly and easily determine anyone's electrical axis." But it wasn't long before people started coming to me with EKGs showing isoelectric complexes in *each* of the three limb leads. They'd say, "This doesn't fit your pattern! Your system stinks." As you can imagine, it was pretty disheartening to hear that kind of feedback.

When I come across something I just can't figure out, I take it to someone who probably can. For this particular dilemma I went to Dr. Gerald Gordon, a cardiologist who has instructed paramedics for many years. I showed him my system, explained its development, and then showed him the EKGs with isoelectric leads I, II, and III. "What is this?" I asked him. He then explained *reniform axis* to me. Instead of traveling linearly through the heart, the cardiac impulses travel a kidney-shaped path.

This kidney-shaped route inscribes isoelectric complexes in each of the limb leads. *Ren* meaning "kidney," a kidney-shaped axis is a reniform axis. So I amended my system to include *six* patterns to memorize in order to determine axis.

Then, after teaching the six pattern method for a year or more, I accidently discovered what I believe to be the genesis of reniform axis. My partner and I were at the residence of a 70-year-old gentleman who had suffered a cardiac arrest. His initial quick-look was asystole. He remained in asystole despite our performance of all the appropriate ACLS protocols. So, after emptying half of our drug box into the patient's IV line, I called my base physician and got the order for a field pronouncement. My partner went out to the other room to do the family notification, while I busied myself cleaning up our mess.

Soon after hearing the piercing cries characteristic of someone just informed that her loved one was dead, my partner came back in and grabbed the Lifepack IV.[*] She said, "His wife's having a little bit of chest pressure. I just want to run a quick strip on her, make sure she's doin' alright." While she went to do that, I finished cleaning up.

When I rejoined my partner, I happened to glance at the EKG she had run on this patient. The EKG showed complexes that were isoelectric in lead I, isoelectric in lead II, and isoelectric in lead III. This woman had a reniform axis. I was excited. I'd never had a patient with a reniform axis! I'd only seen it on EKGs other people had brought to me.

And then I noticed where my partner had placed the electrodes. Right upper chest, left upper chest, and left upper abdomen. So I got out another set of patches and put the electrodes where they were properly meant to be. As it turned out, the woman had a physiologic left axis, *not* a reniform axis.

Since then, when people bring me an EKG showing reniform axis, I've asked them where they placed the electrodes. One hundred percent of the time, so far, the electrodes have been inaccurately placed. This is why I'm not convinced that reniform axis actually exists. It may. Somewhere, sometime, we may come up with clinical evidence showing that the magnetic pull of Uranus and Jupiter opposing each other causes this kidney-shaped electrical stuff—I don't know. I can't say that it's impossible. So, for the sake of completeness, I still include reniform axis when I teach axis determination. But I stress the fact that inaccurately placed electrodes were responsible for *all* the reniform axis EKGs that I have ever seen.

---

[*]For those of you who haven't been around long enough to be familiar with a Lifepack IV, it was a 40-pound EKG unit that was virtually indestructible. It could be dropped down several flights of stairs, picked up, and still successfully used to defibrillate a patient. It also is probably the genesis of the unilateral shoulder hypertrophy you may see on many older paramedics.

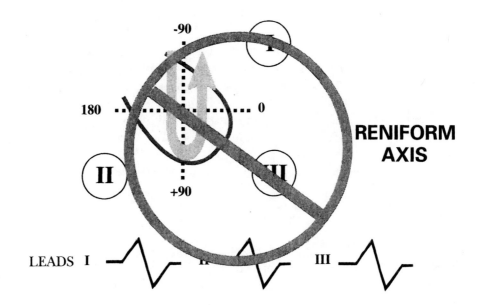

RENIFORM
AXIS

LEADS I   II   III

FIGURE 3.8 An axis created by the kidney-shaped travel of electrical activity through the heart, inscribing isoelectric complexes in leads I, II, and III. *Ren* meaning "kidney," a kidney-shaped axis is a reniform axis.

I think it was Einstein who said, "Never commit to memory anything that can be written down." So in the appendix I have provided you with a collection of figures to photocopy and reduce. The collection includes the chart in Figure 3.9. Tape the reduced copy to your monitor or keep it in your wallet. Each time you run an EKG, run leads I, II, and III. Then just compare the primary direction of each lead's deflection to the chart. It's quick and easy to determine the matching axis pattern. Before too long, you'll discover that you've accidently memorized all of them!

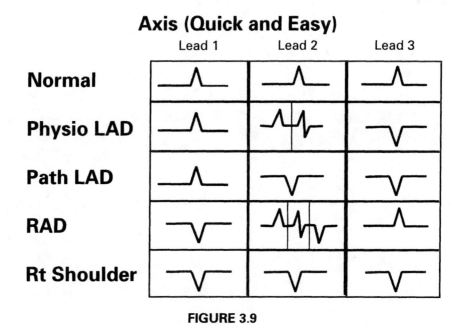

Axis (Quick and Easy)

FIGURE 3.9

SUMMARY

It's easy to include axis determination as part of your routine analysis of every electrocardiogram. Simply attach the limb leads to the *limbs*, run leads I, II, and III, and then monitor your patient in MCL_1. As you will soon learn, axis determination is vitally important to the identification of hemiblocks and is also helpful in the differential diagnosis of wide complex tachycardias. Determination of your patient's axis may help to significantly improve the quality of care you render. It may even prevent accidental mistreatment.

REFERENCE

1. Goldman, Mervin J.: *Principles of Clinical Electrocardiography.* Lange Medical Publications, Los Altos, California, 1982.

CHAPTER **4**

Hemiblocks

Now we are ready to deal with hemiblocks (also called *fascicular* blocks). Although the term *hemiblock* technically should mean "half-a-block," it is universally used to indicate the presence of a block in one of the two major fascicles (divisions) of the heart's left bundle branch, either the anterior fascicle or the posterior fascicle.

People who respond to the mention of axis with moans and groans usually moan and groan even louder in response to the mention of hemiblocks. And EKG instructors who insist that you don't need to know how to determine axis are equally convinced that you don't need to know about hemiblocks. However, hemiblocks are the main *reason* you need to know how to determine axis! Diagnosis of the absence or presence of a hemiblock is, to the greatest extent, determined by the patient's axis. It is my opinion that the inability to determine the presence of a hemiblock has often been the cause of complete heart block when well-intentioned caregivers have improperly administered lidocaine. We'll deal with this inflammatory statement later after I've helped you to understand hemiblocks.

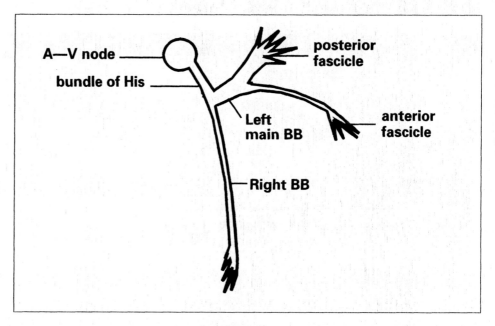

FIGURE 4.1

First, let's review the anatomic structure of the A-V node and bundle branches. As you can see in Figure 4.1, the A-V node connects with the bundle of His, which is about a centimeter long. The His bundle rapidly divides into the right bundle branch and the left main bundle branch. The left main bundle branch is very thick (compared to the right bundle branch), but also very short. It almost immediately divides into an anterior fascicle and a posterior fascicle. There are also usually some fibers that come off the left main bundle branch and innervate the septum directly. The right bundle branch does not have fascicular divisions.

The anterior fascicle is a long, thin structure. Its only blood supply is the left anterior descending coronary artery. The posterior fascicle is shorter and twice as thick and has blood supplied by both the right coronary artery and the left circumflex artery. Because of this, it requires a greater amount of disease to block the posterior fascicle than the anterior fascicle. Therefore, an anterior hemiblock is more common than a posterior hemiblock. Not surprisingly, a posterior hemiblock is much more serious for the patient than an anterior hemiblock.

First, for *any* hemiblock, the duration of the QRS complex must be either within normal limits (less than 0.12 seconds) or it must show a right bundle branch block pattern. If you have a left bundle branch block, *both* fascicles are blocked.

If the patient has a *pathologic* left axis deviation and either a normal QRS complex or a right bundle branch block, the patient has an anterior hemiblock. A patient with a posterior hemiblock will have a right axis deviation and (usually) a right bundle branch block, with no evidence of *right ventricular hypertrophy.*

Okay. Now, I'll explain the previous paragraph and help you to actually *understand* hemiblocks.

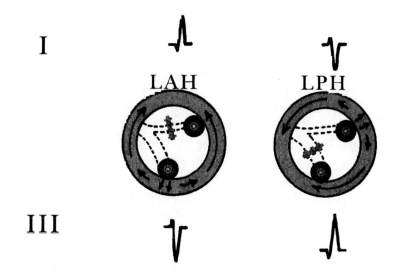

FIGURE 4.2 (Henry J. L. Marriott: *Practical Electrocardiography,* 8th ed., 1988; Williams & Wilkins, Baltimore.)

The posterior fascicle supplies a majority of the inferior wall of the left ventricle. The anterior fascicle supplies innervation to more of the superior wall of the left ventricle.

If the anterior fascicle is blocked, the initial impulse travels toward the bottom half of the ventricle, giving you a little bit of a q wave in lead I and a little bit of an r wave in lead III (LAH diagram of Figure 4.2). The rest of the impulse goes around toward the top part of the ventricles—going toward lead I and inscribing a positive deflection there and going away from lead III and inscribing a negative deflection. This produces the pathologic left axis deviation pattern, with a little q in lead I and a little r in lead III.

So, to diagnose an anterior hemiblock, the first thing you need is a pathologic left axis deviation with either a normal QRS complex or a right bundle branch block. For prehospital purposes, that's all you need to grossly diagnose an anterior hemiblock. (Those who want to be 100 percent sure will look for a little q in lead I and a little r in lead III.)

Exactly the opposite is true for a posterior hemiblock. When the posterior fascicle is blocked, the initial impulse travels to the top part of the left ventricle, producing a little r wave in I and a little q wave in III (LPH diagram of Figure 4.2). Then the impulse travels down and around to the bottom of the ventricles, going away from lead I and toward lead III. This inscribes a right axis deviation pattern with a little r in I and a little q in III.

To diagnose a posterior hemiblock all you need is a right axis deviation with either a normal QRS complex or a right bundle branch block. In fact, because it is difficult to damage the posterior fascicle without also damaging the right bundle branch, a patient with a posterior hemiblock almost always also has a right bundle branch block. If you can see a little r in I and a little q in III, you have confirmed a posterior hemiblock, as long as there is *no evidence of right ventricular hypertrophy.*

What would be the clinical evidence of right ventricular hypertrophy? Jugular venous distension, pedal edema, presacral edema. Those are good indicators of right ventricular hypertrophy. Patients who would commonly have hypertrophy of the right ventricle include some congestive heart failure patients and anyone with asthma, bronchitis, or emphysema. Chronic lung disease causes a compensatory right ventricular hypertrophy in order to push blood through the hypertensive pulmonary veins. In addition, alcoholics frequently have ventricular hypertrophy, secondary to both the cardiomyopathy and hypertension that alcoholism causes.

What does right ventricular hypertrophy look like on the electrocardiogram? The classic combination is an upright complex in MCL_1 and a right axis deviation. Since right ventricular hypertrophy causes a right axis deviation, and right axis deviation is the prime diagnostic finding in posterior hemiblock, it is easy to mistake one for the other.

Now, in the prehospital setting, does a concern about right ventricular hypertrophy make much difference? Not really, because if we suspect a posterior hemiblock, we're going to approach the patient as if he's got it.

Marriott did a small study of 250 patients with acute myocardial infarction. He found that 11 percent of them had an anterior hemiblock alone, 4 percent had an anterior hemiblock with a right bundle branch block, and only 1 percent had a posterior hemiblock with a right bundle branch block. *Nobody* had a posterior hemiblock alone.[1]

Another interesting study involving 3160 patients with myocardial infarction had a grand total of 70 patients (2.22 percent) with a posterior hemiblock. Of those patients, 10 (14 percent) died before they left the hospital. Forty-six of the surviving 60 patients received a follow-up investigation. Twenty-nine (63 percent) had persistent chest pain, 10 (22 percent) had congestive heart failure, and 6 (13 percent) had recurrent AMI. The other 4 were dead within 20 days to 24 months. A posterior fascicular block is a grave prognostic sign.[2]

Figure 4.3 summarizes the criteria used to identify the presence of a left anterior or left posterior hemiblock.

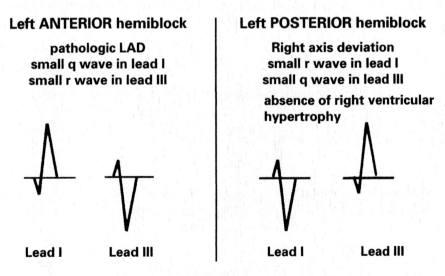

Left ANTERIOR hemiblock

pathologic LAD
small q wave in lead I
small r wave in lead III

Lead I   Lead III

Left POSTERIOR hemiblock

Right axis deviation
small r wave in lead I
small q wave in lead III

absence of right ventricular
hypertrophy

Lead I   Lead III

FIGURE 4.3

I know of only one published case of a posterior hemiblock without a right bundle branch block. Unfortunately, I can't remember the publication or author to acknowledge for the figures accompanying this case. A cardiologist photocopied the figures and article and gave them to me.

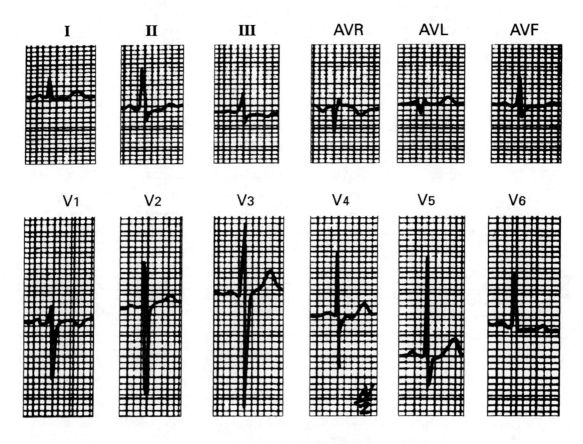

FIGURE 4.4

Figure 4.4 is the EKG of a 32-year-old male before he went into the hospital for some surgery on one of his cardiac valves. You can see that his axis is normal: upright QRS complexes in I, II, and III.

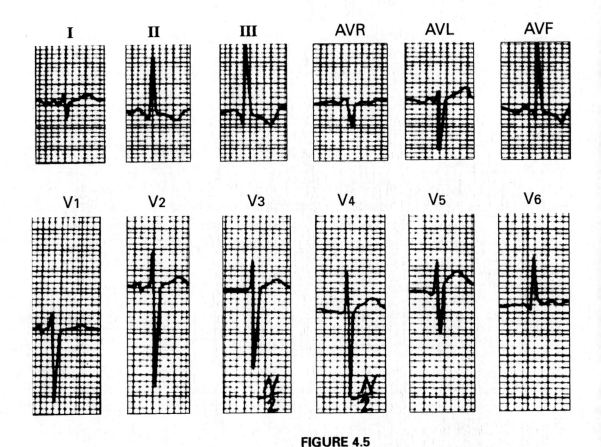

FIGURE 4.5

As you can see in Figure 4.5, which was recorded after the surgery, the lead I complexes are negative, the complexes in leads II and III are positive, and he has a little r in I and a little q in III. He now has a posterior hemiblock without a right bundle branch block. During his valve surgery, the surgeon accidentally cut his posterior fascicle! This is an *iatrogenic* (health care provider-caused) posterior hemiblock. Fortunately for him, this particular posterior hemiblock probably does not represent as grave a prognostic sign as it does in someone with cardiac disease.

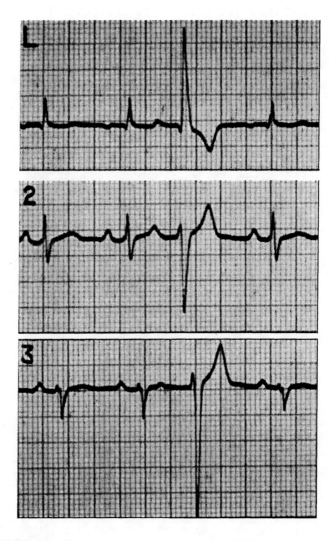

FIGURE 4.6   (Henry J. L. Marriott: *Practical Electrocardiography*, 8th ed., 1988; Williams & Wilkins, Baltimore.)

Figure 4.6 is a series of three concurrent (simultaneously inscribed) EKG strips. It shows aVL (which is very similar to lead I), lead II, and lead III. If you look at the underlying beats represented by the first two and last complexes in each strip, you'll notice that the aVL QRS complexes are upright, lead II's are isoelectric (the same amount above as below), and lead III's are negative. Thus, the underlying rhythm has a physiologic left axis deviation. On the larger, early QRS complexes (the third one on each strip), the aVL QRS complex is upright, while leads II and III show negative QRS complexes. This demonstrates a pathologic left axis deviation. These early complexes are each of premature atrial origin. In aVL the early beats have a little q wave and a tall R wave. There is a little r wave and deep S wave in lead III's early beat. This PAC exhibits an anterior hemiblock aberration.

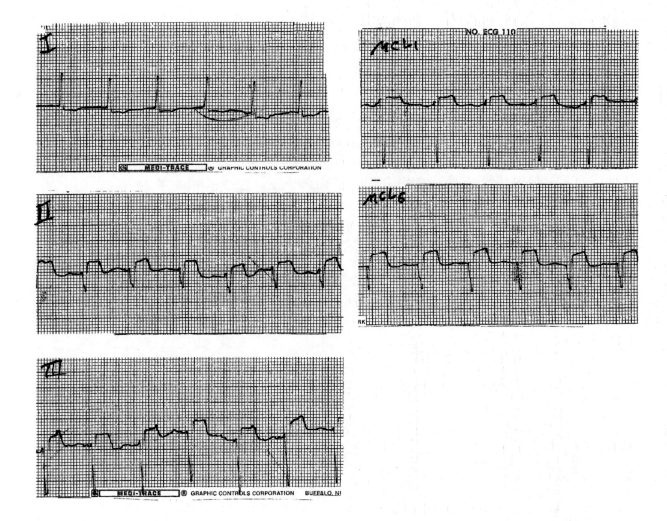

FIGURE 4.7

If you look at the axis in Figure 4.7, lead I is upright and leads II and III are negative, exhibiting a pathologic left axis deviation. The QRS complex measures 0.07 seconds wide, so it is not wide enough to have a bundle branch block. There is a P wave before each QRS complex, and the rate is about 96. So this is a sinus rhythm with a pathologic left axis deviation, indicating the presence of an anterior hemiblock. (The S-T segment elevation in leads II, III, and MCL$_6$ also indicates a possible area of ischemia, a topic discussed in Chapter Eleven.)

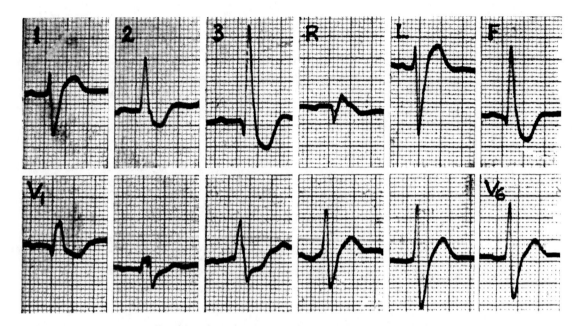

FIGURE 4.8 (Reproduced by permission of Dr. Henry J. L. Marriott, Director of Clinical Research and Education, Rogers Heart Foundation, St. Anthony's Hospital, St. Petersburg, Florida.)

Figure 4.8 is a 12-lead electrocardiogram. You can see that lead I is negative, while leads II and III are upright, indicating right axis deviation. Lead I has a little bit of an r wave, and lead III has a little bit of a q wave. This patient has a posterior hemiblock. The QRS complexes are wide (0.12 or 0.13 seconds wide). If you find the J point in V_1 (which is virtually the same as MCL_1) and draw a line back into the complex, you will find that the triangle points up. This is like a right turn signal, so this indicates a right bundle branch block. This patient has a right bundle branch block, a right axis deviation, and a left posterior fascicular block. Consequently, the only fascicle in this patient's heart that is conducting impulses to the ventricle normally is the anterior fascicle of the left bundle branch. This patient has a very sick heart.

Okay, here comes the "method" behind all the "madness" of this text. Paramedics need to be able to determine axis deviation in order to recognize hemiblocks. And we need to be able to diagnose hemiblocks for the same reason that we must be able to recognize bundle branch blocks and A-V heart blocks. All these blocks assist us to identify patients who are at high risk for developing complete heart block. Certain of these blocks are warning signs or *precursors* to complete heart block.

PRECURSORS TO COMPLETE HEART BLOCK

The first group of precursors to complete heart block are *all* the type II blocks: occasional dropped beats type II, 2:1 block type II, and high-grade A-V block type II. Patients with any of the type II A-V heart blocks are at greater risk for developing complete heart block.

The second group includes patients who have demonstrated disease in both bundle branches. When a patient has a right bundle branch block in his living room, but when you get him to the ambulance he has a left bundle branch block, the patient has demonstrated disease in both bundle branches. This patient is at great risk for developing complete heart block.

The third group are those patients with any *two or more* of the other blocks. Any two or more together. A patient with a prolonged P-R interval and an anterior hemiblock has two blocks and is at higher risk for developing complete heart block. Some other examples:

- Right bundle branch block and an anterior hemiblock
- Right bundle branch block with a posterior hemiblock
- Prolonged P-R interval with an anterior hemiblock
- Prolonged P-R interval with an anterior hemiblock and a right bundle branch block

Any combination of two or more blocks indicates a high risk of going into complete heart block.

But why is it so important to recognize patients who are at high risk

---

Precursors to Complete Heart Block

1. Any type II A-V heart block: occasional dropped beats type II, 2:1 block type II, or high-grade A-V block type II.

2. Any patient demonstrating disease in both bundle branches.

3. Any combination of two or more blocks.

---

for complete heart block? First, you won't be so surprised when they do it! In fact, you'll be ready for it. You'll recognize whether or not your patient is likely to need a pacemaker and whether or not you should prophylactically put the transcutaneous pacer pads on them. Second, you'll know that the administration of lidocaine may precipitate complete heart block. Unless a pacemaker is present, lidocaine is contraindicated in any patient with the precursors to complete heart block![3]

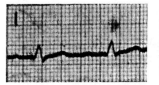 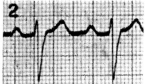 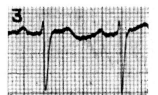 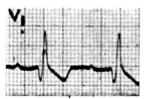

FIGURE 4.9 (Reproduced by permission of Dr. Henry J. L. Marriott, Director of Clinical Research and Education, Rogers Heart Foundation, St. Anthony's Hospital, St. Petersburg, Florida.)

Take a look at Figure 4.9: upright complexes in lead I, negative complexes in leads II and III. What is the axis? Pathologic left axis deviation. What should come to mind? Anterior hemiblock. Note the width of the QRS complexes and look at V_1. Right bundle branch block. What does the P-R interval measure? It's greater than 0.20 seconds. Prolonged P-R interval. When you put it all together, this patient has a prolonged P-R interval, an anterior hemiblock, and a right bundle branch block.

What portion of this patient's electrophysiological anatomy is conducting in a *normal* manner to the ventricles? The posterior left fascicle. That's it. There is delayed conduction from the atria to the ventricles, evidenced by the prolonged P-R interval. And, within the ventricles, both the right bundle branch and anterior left fascicle are already blocked. The posterior fascicle is the only remaining pathway of normal conduction.

Now, what would happen if this patient started having PVCs? Would the people who insist you don't need to know anything about bundle branch blocks, axis, and hemiblocks be concerned about giving lidocaine to this patient? Remember that they will only see the "first-degree heart block" and a wide QRS complex. They will probably not be concerned about administering lidocaine.

What about you? Knowing what you know *now*, would you give this patient lidocaine? I hope not. At least not without a pacemaker in place and ready to go.

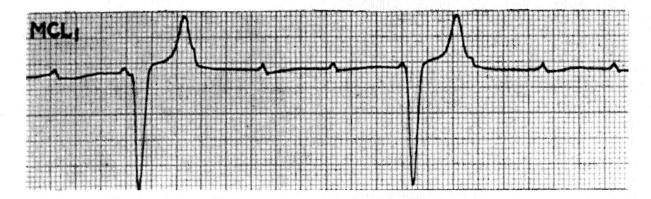

FIGURE 4.10 (Reproduced by permission of Dr. Henry J. L. Marriott, Director of Clinical Research and Education, Rogers Heart Foundation, St. Anthony's Hospital, St. Petersburg, Florida.)

This patient did, in fact, have some PVCs. And, unfortunately, this patient received lidocaine prior to a pacemaker. Figure 4.10 shows what happened after the lidocaine administration. Although the patient certainly was a candidate for a pacemaker before he got the lidocaine, now he is in complete heart block and needs one *much sooner* than he did before!

Figure 4.11 shows this same patient's electrocardiogram after receiving his pacemaker.

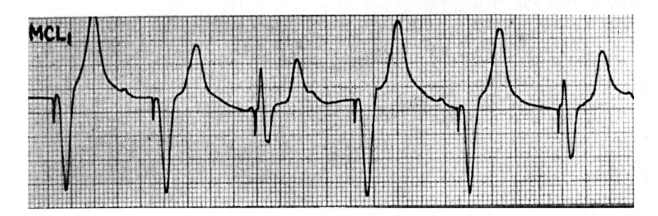

FIGURE 4.11 (Reproduced by permission of Dr. Henry J. L. Marriott, Director of Clinical Research and Education, Rogers Heart Foundation, St. Anthony's Hospital, St. Petersburg, Florida.)

SUMMARY

Now you know why it is essential to understand the reclassification of A-V blocks: to identify which bundle branch is blocked and to be able to determine axis and diagnose hemiblocks. People who believe that they "don't need to know these things" won't be able to properly anticipate the evolution of their patients' diseases and are putting those patients at significant risk for injury because of inappropriate treatment.

Understanding the reclassification of A-V blocks, bundle branch blocks, axis determination, and hemiblocks allows you to predict your patient's prognosis with some degree of accuracy. Will your patient need a pacemaker? Should you apply the transcutaneous pacer pads prophylactically? Is it safe to give lidocaine? What is your return mode—do you need to use lights and sirens? And where will you take the patient—to any old health care institution or to a hospital with a cath-lab, able to install a pacemaker? You should now be well equipped to answer *all* these questions.

REFERENCES

1. Marriott, H. J. L., and Hogan, P.: Hemiblock in acute myocardial infarction. *Chest* 1970:58, 342–4.

2. Lewin, R. F., et al.: Right axis deviation in acute myocardial infarction. Clinical significance, hospital evolution, and long-term follow-up. *Chest* 1984:85(4), 489–93.

3. *Drug Facts and Comparisons*, J.B. Lippincott Co., St. Louis, MO, May 1992, pp. 146f–i.

CHAPTER **5**

Case *Studies*

The purpose of this chapter is to review the things we've learned so far: the reclassification of A-V blocks, identification of bundle branch blocks, electrical axis determination, diagnosis of hemiblocks, and identification of the precursors to complete heart block. And because I can't help myself, I'll throw in little bits of extra information as we go along.

A standard approach to interpreting or "reading" electrocardiograms might be this:

- Place electrodes properly to ensure an accurate EKG.

- Run a strip showing leads I, II, III, and MCL_1.

- Scan the QRS rate. Is it fast, slow, or within normal limits?

- Scan for any patterns of regularity or irregularity. Are there groups of beats?

- Determine the axis.

- Look at the width of the QRS complexes. Are they within normal limits, or is a bundle branch blocked?

- Observe the P waves. Are there any? If so, what is their relationship to the QRS complexes? Do they have one? How long is the P-R interval?

- After that, you can identify dysrhythmias, infarction patterns, and all that other stuff!

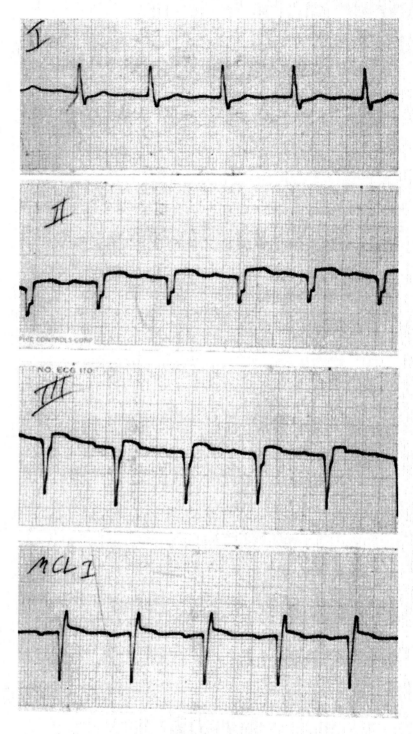

FIGURE 5.1

Figure 5.1 is the EKG of a 52-year-old male who had a syncopal episode after playing tennis on a hot summer day. I'll call him Bob. When we arrived, Bob was walking around gathering up his tennis balls, his racket, and getting ready to leave. He had theater tickets for the evening and was in a rush to get home to shower. His friends had called 911 when he passed out, but he was "fine" now and certainly wasn't interested in seeing us! When I convinced him that we could check him out quickly, Bob submitted to an exam.

Bob was asymptomatic. He had no trauma from the syncopal episode and insisted that he "didn't even really pass all the way out." Bob estimated he had played tennis for almost two hours prior to the incident and "probably didn't drink enough water."

Looking at Figure 5.1, what is evident on Bob's EKG? He's got a sinus rhythm with a prolonged P-R interval. The rhythm is regular. There is no ectopy. The QRS complexes in lead I are primarily positive, but in II and III the QRS complexes are primarily negative. Hold that up to your handy chart, and what is Bob's axis? Pathologic left axis deviation.

The QRS complexes are wide, so look at MCL_1 to determine which bundle branch is blocked. Draw in your arrow from the J point if you need to, and the arrow points up. Turn signal goes up for a right turn. Right bundle branch block.

Bob has a pathologic left axis deviation with a right bundle branch block; what does that tell us? He's got a left anterior hemiblock. Although we can't clearly see a little q in I or a little r in III, in the prehospital setting it still needs to be approached as though there was a left anterior hemiblock present.

So put it all together: sinus rhythm, prolonged P-R interval, right bundle branch block, and left anterior hemiblock. Should Bob drive home, take a shower, and get ready to go to the theater? I don't think so. His electrocardiogram identifies him as being at high risk for complete heart block. In fact, a transient episode of a high-grade or complete heart block may have been the cause of his syncopal episode. If he has another episode of this, there is no guarantee that it will be *transient* again.

Getting Bob to go to the hospital was probably one of the hardest "sells" of my career. I think it got to the point where my partner actually drew up a last will and testament for him to sign! At last we convinced him how serious the consequences could be if he didn't go. While in the emergency room, he went into complete heart block with significant hypoperfusion. His pressure dropped to 60 systolic, and he received a permanent pacemaker.

This is another example of why paramedics need to understand more than just "lead II cardiology." A paramedic who couldn't recognize the seriousness of Bob's EKG would have probably let him go home.

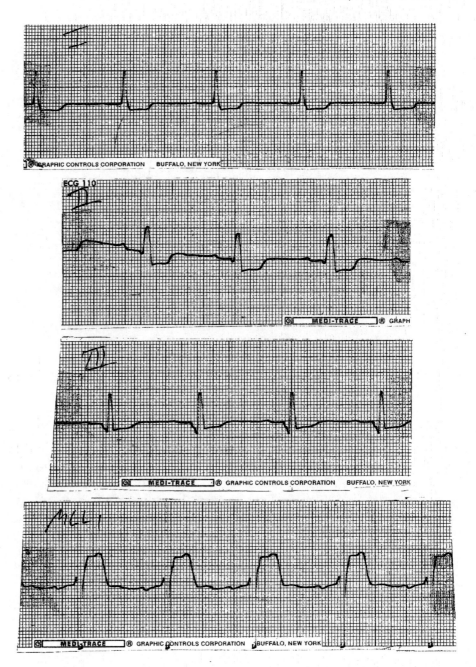

FIGURE 5.2

In Figure 5.2 the rhythm is regular, and there is no ectopy. The rate is about 60 to 64 per minute. What is the axis? Upright, upright, upright—positive deflections in leads I, II, and III. Normal axis.

Now, what is the measurement of the QRS complexes? Remember to find a QRS with the clearest beginning and end. In this case, that would be one of the complexes in lead III. Measure that one, compare it to the other leads, and you can see that it is consistently about 0.14 seconds. There is a bundle branch block.

Which bundle branch is blocked? Look at MCL_1. If you have difficulty deciding where the J point is, remember the measurement you took in lead III and apply it here. Draw in your little arrow. Turn signal down for a left turn. Left bundle branch block.

Figure 5.2 is a sinus rhythm. You can clearly see P waves in lead II and MCL_1 and can then identify them in leads I and III. What is the measurement of the P-R interval? It's greater than 0.20 seconds, so its a prolonged P-R interval.

Something noteworthy about this strip is the S-T elevation in MCL_1. Later in this text we'll discuss cardiac ischemia and its manifestations on the electrocardiogram. For now, just let me say that S-T changes are what should make us suspect cardiac ischemia. However, a left bundle branch block can *cause* S-T elevation in the right chest leads (of which MCL_1 is one). Consequently, it is difficult—although not impossible—to diagnose cardiac ischemia in the presence of a left bundle branch block.

But, back to our assessment of Figure 5.2. Put it all together: sinus rhythm, regular, no ectopy, prolonged P-R interval, normal axis, and a left bundle branch block. Does this patient fit into any of the groups of precursors to complete heart block? There is no high-grade or type II block present. We have no evidence of disease in both bundle branches. But there is the presence of two or more of the "other" blocks. A prolonged P-R interval and a left bundle branch block. So this patient has a risk of developing complete heart block.

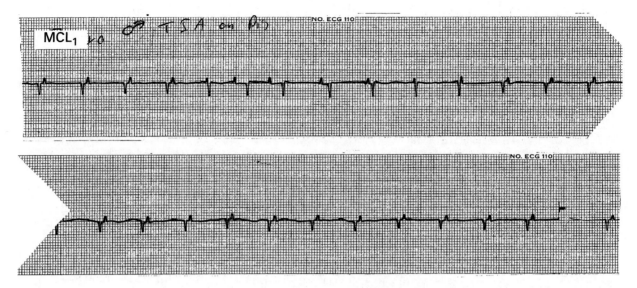

FIGURE 5.3

The EKG in Figure 5.3 is the continuous MCL$_1$ strip of a 74-year-old male whom I will call Mr. Jones. He had a sudden onset of left-sided paralysis and inability to speak. We initiated oxygen by nasal cannula, hooked up the monitor, and were in the process of drawing blood and starting an IV when his neurologic deficits cleared up. Mr. Jones told us he'd been trying to talk to us, but couldn't move, and "it's all better now!" Mr. Jones had apparently suffered a transient ischemic attack. Now that he could speak, Mr. Jones described some nausea and vomiting prior to the episode and told us he was currently taking digitalis for his "heart problem."

I don't have leads I, II, and III for Mr. Jones, so we'll forego the axis determination. What is his rhythm? It's confusing, that's what. So pick it apart.

It's easy to see that this certainly isn't a "normal sinus rhythm." It is grossly regular, though, and has no apparent ectopy. The rate is around 100 and the pointy, little positive deflections are dissociated from the pointy, longer negative deflections. You can clearly see the dissociation in the center of the top strip where the rate altered for a moment. Mr. Jones had taken a deep breath at that particular point in time. That clues you in to the fact that the pointy, little positive deflections are atrial impulses. The pointy, longer negative deflections are Mr. Jones's QRS complexes.

With a rate of 100, QRS complexes measuring less than 0.12 seconds, and A-V dissociation, what is Mr. Jones's EKG? Block–acceleration–dissociation with a junctional escape rhythm. There are plenty of atrial impulses that should conduct, but don't. There is dissociation between the atria and ventricles. And the junction is providing an accelerated escape rhythm that is greater than 45 per minute. Because the atria and ventricles happen to have the same rate, this strip can be described as having an *isorhythmic* A-V dissociation.

I wanted to include this strip because it illustrates a typical digitalis-type rhythm. It's bizarre. It reminds me of what a cardiologist once told me about digitalis. He said, "If you've got a patient with a bizarre EKG and they're *not* on digitalis, they probably should be. And if you've got a patient with a bizarre EKG and they're *on* digitalis, they are probably on too much of it!"

Digitalis is a wonderful drug—don't get me wrong! It's useful for congestive heart failure, atrial fibrillation, atrial flutter, and sometimes for paroxysmal atrial tachycardia.[1] Like most drugs, digitalis is marketed under a number of different names: Digoxin, Digitoxin, Crystodigin, Lanoxin, and Lanoxicaps. But at least the drug manufacturers have done us the unusual favor of making them all sound enough alike so that we can recognize a digitalis medication.

The next case study involves a 70-year-old male who dialed 911 because he had some chest pain. But before we discuss this case and its electrocardiogram, I want to share some techniques for patient interview techniques that I feel are pretty important.

When you get dispatched to "elderly male with chest pain," what words are often included in your initial contact with the patient? "Good morning. I'm Debbie, a paramedic with General Hospital's ambulance service. Are you the person having chest pain?" Debbie has appropriately introduced herself, but inappropriately limited the patient's description of the problem to "chest pain." Many patients consider the sensation in their chest to be "discomfort" or "tightness" or "heaviness." An open-ended question like "What seems to be wrong today?" yields clearer, more patient-specific information.

When you have a patient who complains about chest discomfort of any kind, what do you want to know about it? One of the first things I like to know is, has the patient had this discomfort before? "Yes, I've had three heart attacks."

The key question when someone tells you they've had a "heart attack" is this, "How long were you in the hospital?" If they answer, "Oh! All afternoon, it was terrible!" you can be fairly sure that the patient wasn't discharged with the diagnosis of AMI. And although you still can't discount the fact that they have had chest discomfort in the past and are having it now, you might comfortably discount the previous history of a "heart attack." However, if their response is, "Well, I was in the CCU for two weeks, and then they moved me to a regular floor for another week or so," you immediately know that this patient has a cardiac history that is seriously significant.

There is a wide variety of questions important to the investigation of chest discomfort. Is this chest discomfort the same as before or is it different? If it's different, *how* is it different? What were you doing when it started? What have you done to make it better? And then there's the *ten scale*. "On a scale of one to ten, ten being the worst pain you've ever felt, where would you rate this discomfort?" "Oh! It's a twelve!" Whatever number the patient replies with, there is one more piece of information that you need to make this ten scale meaningful. What *is* the worst pain you've ever felt? If the worst pain Mr. Smith has ever had is a hangnail, the rating of twelve for his chest discomfort isn't that impressive. But if the worst pain he's ever had was a kidney stone the size of a cue ball, twelve is incredible pain. You need to have a reference as to the patient's worst pain to be able to use the ten scale meaningfully.

How long have you had this discomfort? *Where* is the discomfort? The best locater of chest discomfort is to have the patient use one finger to draw a circle around it.

Let's discuss one common question: "Does the pain go anywhere?" People ask that question when trying to determine whether or not the chest discomfort radiates. Well, if the patient's left arm has been aching for two days, but his chest discomfort is new, how will he answer that question? "No, it doesn't go anywhere." He had discomfort in his arm *first,* so he may not associate it with the discomfort in his chest. If you want to determine whether the patient has radiating pain, use the words "Do you hurt anywhere else?" "Yes, my left arm has been aching for a couple of days now."

How do you ask about the *quality* of chest pain? "Describe your chest pain for me." "Well, it's pain. You know, pain?" A typical response is then to ask "Is the pain sharp or dull?" This is a bad question. If your patient is experiencing "tearing" chest pain and you only provide a choice of "sharp" or "dull," you may miss a critical diagnostic clue, one that could help you to identify a dissecting aortic aneurysm (which needs a significantly different approach to treatment and management than does a myocardial infarction). Instead of suggesting specific pain descriptions, cue the patient to "describe your pain in your own words."

If your patient is unable to spontaneously give you a description of the quality of the discomfort, it's sometimes helpful to ask, "What would I have to *do* to you to create this same kind of discomfort?" This may bring answers like, "You'd have to tear me in half," or "set me on fire," or "punch me in the chest," or "stab me," and so on. This is a much less suggestive approach for determining the quality of discomfort.

Of course, you want to ask about associated complaints such as nausea, vomiting (how many times? what did it look like?), and sweating.

How do you ask about shortness of breath? Again, don't use words that lead the patient on: "Are you short of breath?" Anyone having an emergency, when asked if they are "short of breath" will concentrate on their breathing and usually decide, "Yeah, I guess I am!" If you want to know how well they are breathing ask them, "How's your breathing?" And if they say, "My breathing's fine," leave it alone! Some people have no impulse control and will continue to ask the patient, "You're sure you aren't having trouble breathing?" If a patient says their breathing is fine, it's fine—from a historical perspective. If you don't believe their answer, then describe what you see and ask, "Is this 'normal' for you?"

Asking all patients about their medications is vital because this information both provides important clues to the patient's past medical history and assists your evaluation of the current complaint. But pay attention to *how* you ask about medications. Some people ask, "Do you take medications prescribed by a doctor?" In response to that question, patients will be unlikely to report the over-the-counter medications they take, such as daily aspirin. Another trap is to ask a patient, "What medications do you take every day?" The patient will probably tell you exactly that, but may *not* tell you about the occasional nitroglycerin tablet, or the immunosuppressant therapy they get every other day, or the injections of antipsychotic medication they get every three or four weeks.

Ask the patient, "What medications do you take?" If there are several, they sometimes tend to stop reciting them before the list is completed. Or they forget one or two of them. Keep pressing, "What *other* medications do you take?" until you're sure the list is thorough.

Then there are the patients who don't take certain medications they're supposed to, so they don't tell you about them unless you ask, "Are there medications you're supposed to be taking but aren't?" You may or may not get an honest answer to that one. Many people find the odor and taste of potassium extremely offensive. They keep taking their Lasix, but stop taking the potassium. This is something you need to know!

Finally, "Are you taking your medications the *way* you're supposed to?" They may have them, but if they aren't taking the medications as directed, they won't be receiving the optimal effect.

Medication Questions

1. What medications do you take?

2. What *other* medications do you take?

3. Are there medications you're supposed to be taking but aren't?

4. Are you taking your medications the way you're supposed to?

Let's look at one more case study. A 70-year-old male—let's call him Mr. Sanchez, dialed 911 because he had some chest pain (and *he* called it "pain").

"Have you had this pain before?"

"Yes, I have. I had a heart attack last year about this time."

"How long were you in the hospital?"

"Oh, I spent about a week in the CCU before they put me in a regular room. And then I had to go back to the CCU unit. So, altogether, about three weeks."

"Is this chest pain the same as before or is it different?"

"It's about the same."

"Mr. Sanchez, do you hurt anywhere else?"

"Well, my left shoulder has been bothering me for a couple of days."

"Describe the chest pain for me, Mr. Sanchez, what does it feel like?"

"Oh, I don't know, sort of like a vise across my chest."

"How's your breathing?"

"My breathing's okay, but the pain is so bad that I don't feel like I'm getting enough air!"

Now, even without knowing Mr. Sanchez's medications or any other associated complaints, we have a reasonable idea as to whether Mr. Sanchez's chest pain is cardiac in nature.

What does his EKG show (Figure 5.4)? His sinus rhythm is regular except for the PACs or PJCs captured in lead I. He doesn't appear to have any ventricular ectopy. He has a pathologic left axis deviation with QRS complexes within normal limits. Left anterior hemiblock. It's hard to see little q waves in lead I, but he certainly has little r waves in lead III. His P-R interval looks to be about 0.20 seconds, so its "borderline" but within normal limits.

If Mr. Sanchez developed a need for lidocaine, would you be comfortable administering it? I think so. Although his P-R interval is close to being prolonged, it's not. The only block he has is an anterior hemiblock. He doesn't fit into any of the precursor groups for complete heart block.

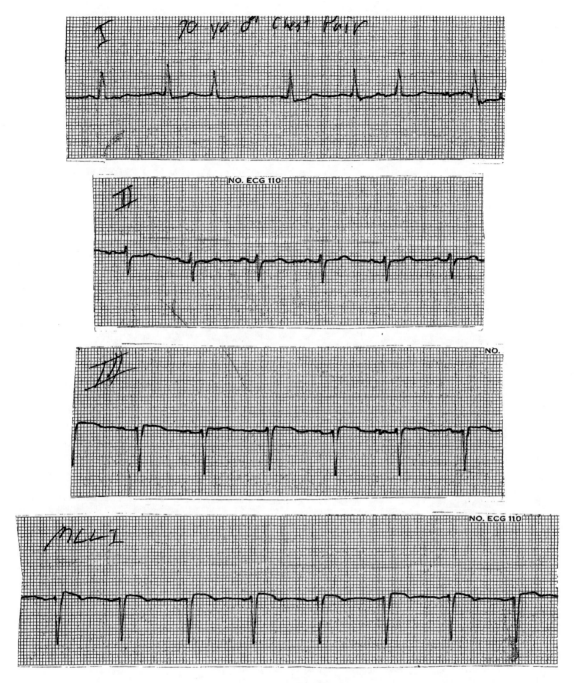

FIGURE 5.4

REFERENCE

1. *Drug Facts and Comparisons,* J. B. Lippincott Co., St. Louis, MO, October 1988; digitalis, pp. 141–141f.

CHAPTER 6

Electrophysiology and Effects of Medication

In order to understand the effects of the medications we administer to patients, we need to review the electrophysiology of cell function. The first thing to brush up on is *action potential.* Action potential refers to the electrical changes that occur when a cell is stimulated. This directly corresponds to depolarization and repolarization of working muscle cells and pacemaker cells.

Working muscle cells are those responsible for contraction of muscles. Pacemaker cells make up the system that activates or fires the muscle cells.

Depolarization is defined as the process by which muscle fibers are stimulated to contract. This is accomplished by the alteration of the electrical charge of a cell through changes in electrolyte concentrations across the cell membrane. Repolarization is the process by which cells reestablish internal negativity and are readied for another round of stimulation—a return to the resting or polarized state.

First, let's look at a cell in the resting state and review its electrolyte components. Chemical pumps in a cell's membrane control cell wall permeability and maintain certain concentrations of electrolytes within and without the cell. Sodium and calcium are primarily extracellular electrolytes. Potassium is the primary intracellular electrolyte. The resting (polarized) cell is normally more electrically negative inside the cell wall than outside, -90 millivolts (mV) in working muscle cells. This resting membrane state of a working muscle cell is represented by the phase 4 portion of Figure 6.1.

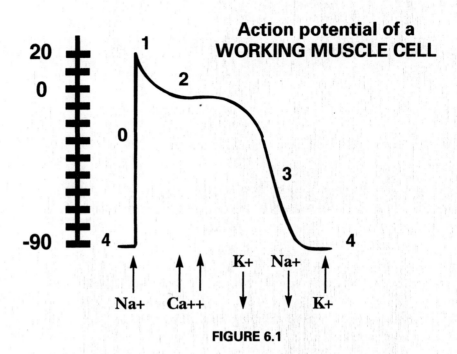

FIGURE 6.1

A working muscle cell can't fire all by itself, so the first phase is when something stimulates the cell from outside. Electrical stimulation ("firing") of a cell membrane changes its permeability to sodium. This means there is then a very rapid influx of sodium, referred to as the "fast channel," causing the cell to become more positive. This rapid influx of sodium into the cell is represented in Figure 6.1 by the high spike of phase 0 to 1.

Then the sodium channel is shut off and the calcium channel is opened, creating the plateau phase, or phase 2 portion of Figure 6.1. Calcium enters the cell more slowly than sodium, via a "slow channel." Medicines such as Verapamil and Cardizem are slow channel calcium blockers. They affect action potential during the plateau phase.

Phase 3 of the action potential occurs when potassium leaks out of the cell. Toward the bottom of phase 3, sodium is pumped out of the cell and potassium returns. The cell can then return to the resting state before starting all over again. That's basically the way it works in muscle cells throughout your body.

Pacemaker cells, in the SA and AV node, have the property of automaticity. They are capable of self-initiated depolarization ("firing"). The ability to fire on their own gives pacemaker cells the property of automaticity. If you were to cut out my biceps muscle and lay it on a table, you'd have a bloody looking biceps lying there in front of you doing absolutely nothing. This is because none of the cells in my biceps have the property of automaticity. But if you were to cut out my heart and lay it on a table, it would continue to try to pump blood for a few moments.

Pacemaker cells have a slightly different action potential. First, they don't start out as negative as the working muscle cells (-70 mV versus -90 mV). Second, the action potential uses calcium; sodium does not play a part in it.

Action potential of a
PACEMAKER CELL

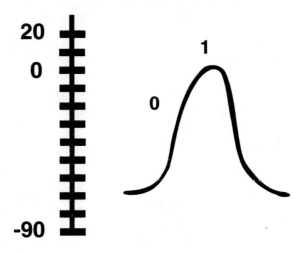

FIGURE 6.2

Consequently, what you get is a slow, upward-sloping phase 0 (Figure 6.2) while potassium slowly leaks out. When enough potassium leaks out and the cell reaches a critical level (phase 1), the cell fires.

There are several aspects of this slow-channel, calcium-mediated action potential that affect the rate of cell firing. The first is the *resting membrane potential*, as seen in Figure 6.3.

RESTING MEMBRANE
POTENTIAL

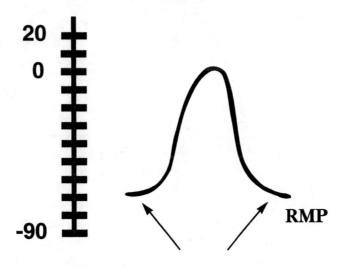

FIGURE 6.3

Again, although a working muscle cell has a resting membrane potential of -90, the resting potential of a pacemaker cell is less negative, about -70. Changes in either resting membrane potential also change the firing rate (Figure 6.4). For example, if you lower the resting membrane potential (making it more negative), it takes longer for the phase 0 slope to reach the threshold where it can fire. Consequently, the next impulse would be delayed and the heart rate would be slowed. Conversely, if you raise the resting membrane potential (making it less negative), it reaches the firing threshold sooner, resulting in another impulse earlier. This produces a faster heart rate.

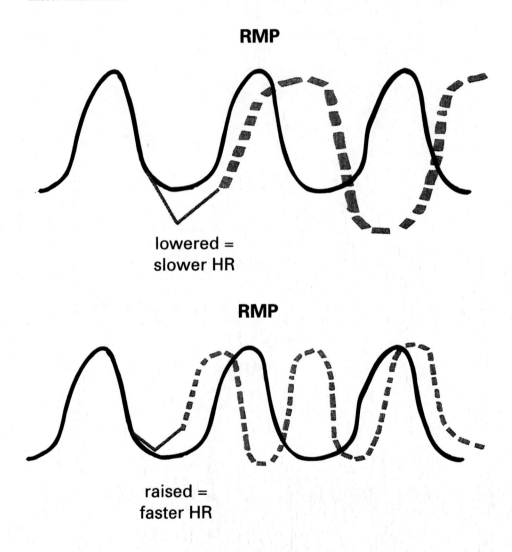

RMP

lowered =
slower HR

RMP

raised =
faster HR

FIGURE 6.4

The next rate-related aspect of the slow-channel (calcium) action potential is the *slope of diastolic depolarization* (Figure 6.5). The slope of diastolic depolarization refers to the slope that begins at the most negative point of the action potential (phase 4), and extends until it reaches the firing threshold (phase 1). This is the phase 0 slope, when potassium is slowly leaking from the cell.

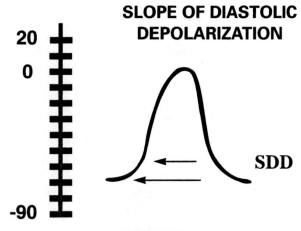

FIGURE 6.5

As with altering the resting membrane potential, if the angle of this slope is changed, the heart rate is changed (Figure 6.6). If the slope of diastolic depolarization is made flatter, it takes longer to reach firing threshold. The next impulse will be delayed, and a slower heart rate will occur, If the slope of diastolic depolarization is made steeper, the firing threshold is reached sooner, thereby increasing the rate of impulse formation.

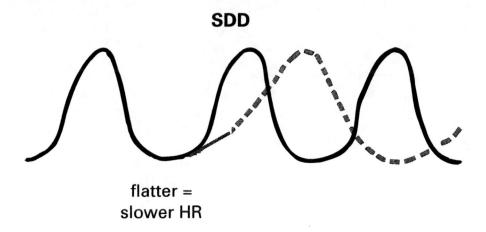

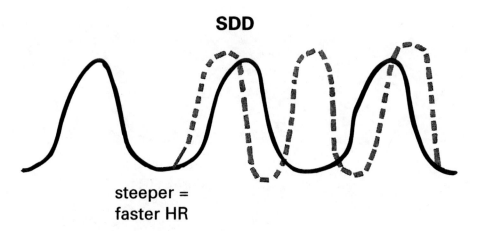

FIGURE 6.6

The last aspect of the slow-channel action potential that can affect heart rate is the *threshold potential* (Figure 6.7). The threshold potential is the point where the cell fires, or phase 1.

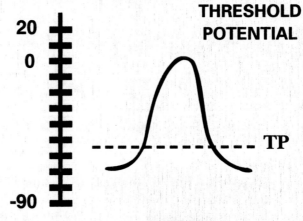

FIGURE 6.7

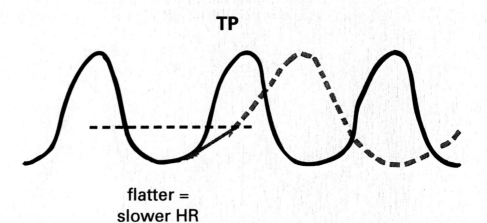

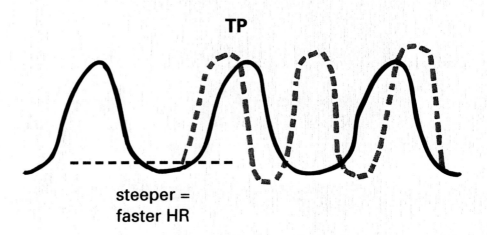

FIGURE 6.8

As you can see in Figure 6.8, if you raise the threshold potential, it takes longer for the slope of diastolic depolarization to reach the firing point. Therefore, the heart rate becomes slower. If you lower the threshold potential, the firing point is reached sooner, and a faster heart rate occurs.

Chemicals and medications that alter heart rate do so by altering one or more of these three aspects of the slow-channel action potential of pacemaker cells. For instance, vagal maneuvers, such as carotid sinus massage, slow the heart rate by stimulating the release of acetylcholine. Acetylcholine affects all three aspects of the slow-channel action potential (Figure 6.9): it lowers the resting membrane potential, it flattens the slope of diastolic depolarization, and it raises the threshold potential. Therefore, impulse formation slows way down. That is the goal when you are trying to convert a supraventricular tachycardia.

ACETYLCHOLINE

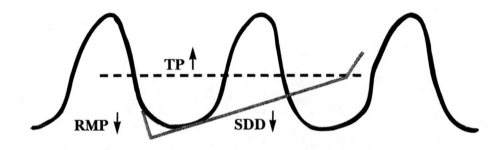

FIGURE 6.9

Epinephrine also affects all three aspects, but in exactly the opposite manner (Figure 6.10). If you stimulate the release of epinephrine (or administer it by injection), you raise the resting membrane potential, make the slope of diastolic depolarization steeper, and decrease the threshold potential. This is how epinephrine increases the heart rate.

EPINEPHRINE

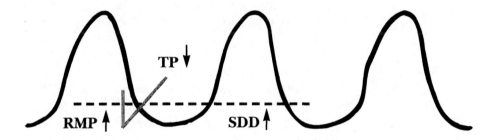

FIGURE 6.10

There are a few other important concepts to understand when reviewing electrophysiology and the effects of medications. One of these is *conduction velocity*. Conduction velocity is the amount of force an action potential is able to pass on to the next cell.

Conduction velocity is measured from the depth of the resting membrane potential (the most negative point of the cell's action potential) to the top of the action potential's slope (the most positive point). As you can see in Figure 6.11, the conduction velocity of a working muscle cell is much greater than that of a pacemaker cell.

CONDUCTION VELOCITY

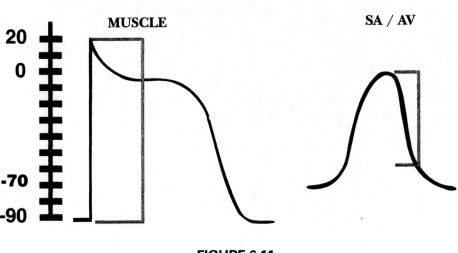

FIGURE 6.11

The next concept to review is *refractory periods*. There are two: *absolute* and *relative*. The absolute refractory period describes the period of time immediately following the firing of an impulse where *no* amount of stimulus will produce another impulse. Not enough of the cell has repolarized, making the cell physically unable to respond to any type of stimulus. The relative refractory period describes the period of time following an impulse when enough repolarization has occurred to allow another stimulus to depolarize (fire) the cell prematurely (Figure 6.12).

Years ago, when first developing my cardiology workshop, I searched and searched for a better way of describing action potentials, conduction velocity, refractory periods, and how to tie them all together. Then a pharmacology professor from Tufts University explained it in a way I could relate to. He said, "All of this is just like flushing a toilet!" Think about it. Picture a toilet (or take this book and go sit on the throne as you continue reading). The tank is full of water. When you push the handle you get a nice big flush. Right after you've pushed the handle though, there's a period of time when you can push the handle all you want but not get the toilet to flush. Not enough water has returned to the tank. That is the absolute refractory period of a toilet flush. If you wait a bit, the tank starts to fill a little more. At a certain point, even though the tank hasn't completely refilled, you can push the handle and get a little flush—a premature flush. That is the relative refractory period of a toilet flush.

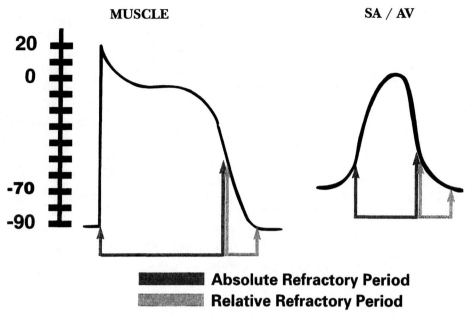

FIGURE 6.12

Notice the difference in the conduction velocity of these flushes. The conduction velocity of a full tank is much greater than that of a partially full tank. Therefore, when you push the handle of a full tank, you get a great big flush, but when you push the handle of a partially full tank you only get a little flush. This exactly corresponds to the conduction velocity differences between a fully repolarized cell and a partially repolarized cell when they are stimulated.

Remember that we're talking about conduction velocity and force of conduction. We're not talking about the force of *contraction* in the heart. It's easy to get confused and assume that a big flush will give you a big contraction. That isn't always so. And that's why it's so important to treat the patient, not the monitor!

ARRHYTHMIAGENESIS

Our next subject is arrhythmiagenesis, the originating cause of arrhythmias. Specifically, we are going to discuss the arrhythmiagenesis of ventricular tachyarrhythmias. Along with this, we are going to briefly discuss lidocaine and its effects on ventricular ectopy and arrhythmias.

There are two well-documented theories as to the origin of ventricular arrhythmias and another theory that remains hypothetical. The first theory is one that most people are familiar with: *enhanced automaticity*.

Picture the SA node firing along as usual when, for some reason, an area of the ventricles develops an irritable site and fires a premature impulse. On the EKG, this irritable impulse would appear as a PVC. If this irritable site continues to fire impulses and attains a rate faster than that of the SA node, it becomes a site of enhanced automaticity and can take over the pacing of the heart. At this point the SA node will stop firing and the EKG will show ventricular tachycardia.

This is not to be confused with a ventricular escape mechanism. A sinus bradycardia that slows down to a rate of 40 (without the atria or junction picking up the pacemaker responsibilities) may be overridden, to the patient's benefit, by a more rapid idioventricular escape mechanism. Enhanced automaticity refers to a pacemaker site other than the SA node that overtakes a rhythm that is operating within normal rate limits.

What happens when you administer lidocaine to a person with an enhanced automaticity arrhythmia? Lidocaine lowers the resting membrane potential (Figure 6.4), makes the slope of diastolic depolarization flatter (Figure 6.6), and raises the threshold potential (Figure 6.8).[1] All this affects the irritable site of enhanced automaticity, thus slowing it down until the SA node can resume its normal rate of fire. This is what is referred to when lidocaine is said to "suppress irritability."

The second theory is one that is probably responsible for the majority of tachyarrhythmias: *reentry*.

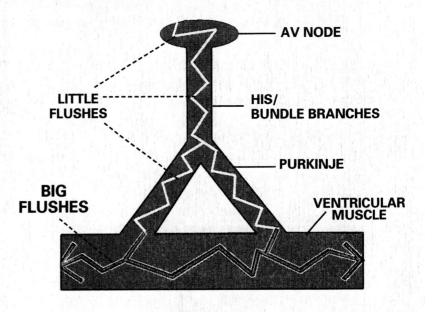

FIGURE 6.13

Normally, impulses from the SA node travel through the A-V junction into the bundle branches and then split and divide through the ventricular conduction pathways until they reach the ventricular wall and fire the muscle (Figure 6.13). Now, using our toilet analogy, compare the impulses that are generated by pacemaker cells and travel the conduction pathways to impulses generated by the responding ventricular muscle cells. Would the pacemaker impulses be considered "big flushes" or "little flushes"? They are little flushes! Remember, the action potential of pacemaker cells is created by low-velocity slow-channel conduction (Figure 6.2). Working muscle cell action potentials are created by a fast channel and have a greater velocity of conduction (Figure 6.1). So what happens when the little flush of a pacemaker impulse gets to the ventricular wall? A big flush of working muscle response occurs!

Now, let's say that someone develops an area of ischemia in one ventricle. Ischemic tissue conducts pacemaker impulses very poorly. In fact, ischemic tissue tends to block them. It takes a strong impulse to travel through ischemic tissue. In Figure 6.14 you can see that pacemaker impulses will travel normally down the nonischemic pathways, but do not have the strength to penetrate the ischemic area. The tissue beyond this block does not get fired and remains in the resting, fully polarized state.

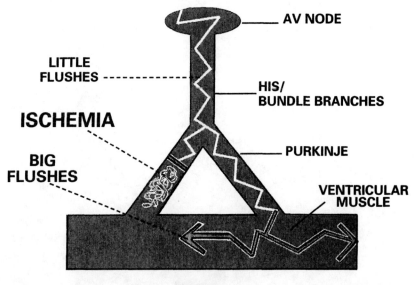

FIGURE 6.14

The pacemaker impulses still reach the ventricular wall via the nonischemic pathways and fire the ventricles. This produces the big flush of ventricular muscle response. And when impulses from this big flush find the unfired tissue of the blocked branch, they fire it in a retrograde direction and trigger its depolarization (Figure 6.15)

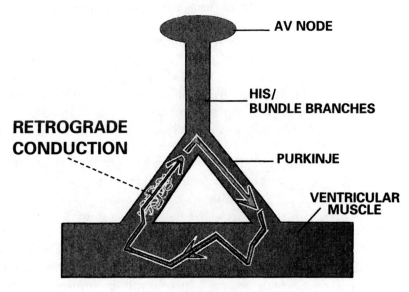

FIGURE 6.15

The big flushes that are traveling retrograde toward the ischemic block are powerful enough to cross the ischemic tissue. And when they reach the other side of the ischemic block, if the tissue they encounter is in its absolute refractory period, the impulses will be unable to travel any further. But if this tissue has had enough time to reach its relative refractory period or has completely repolarized, the tissue will fire prematurely. If this happens once, it's called a PVC. If the circuit continues, as in Figure 6.16, it's called ventricular tachycardia.

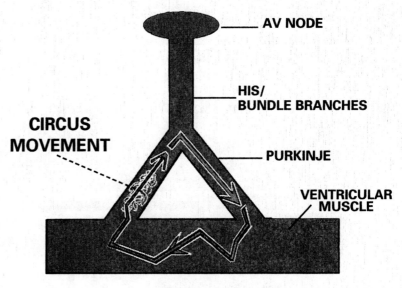

FIGURE 6.16

This is called a *unidirectional* block and is the genesis of the reentry mechanism that produces ventricular tachycardia. This block is called unidirectional because it only blocks the impulses from one direction (the ones from above, the "little flushes"), but allows the retrograde impulses coming from the ventricular wall (the big flushes) to penetrate and reenter the previously fired circuit.

How does lidocaine affect reentry arrhythmias? Well, lidocaine can be considered a myocardial-membranous poison. When it reaches the ischemic area that is too "sick" to conduct pacemaker impulses, lidocaine makes that area a little bit sicker. In fact, it makes the area so sick that it can no longer conduct impulses coming from the ventricular muscle either. Lidocaine takes a unidirectional block and makes it *bi*directional (Figure 6.17). If the ischemic block was producing PVCs, the PVCs are stopped. If ventricular tachycardia was produced by the ischemic block, the ventricular tachycardia is stopped.

Something to keep in mind, however, is that lidocaine goes *everywhere* in the heart—not just to one specific point of ischemia. And lidocaine, being a myocardial-membranous poison, can take a healthy area of the heart and make it just a little bit sick. In this way, lidocaine can actually create a unidirectional block. In fact, lidocaine can cause any of the arrhythmias for which its administration is indicated!

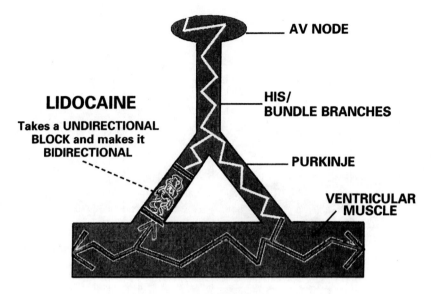

FIGURE 6.17

　　Let's say you have a patient throwing 10 or 12 PVCs a minute and you give him lidocaine. The PVCs diminish to 5 or 6 a minute. Then you hang a lidocaine drip. But soon the PVCs increase to 18 per minute! There is no way, that I know of, to tell whether the patient's original problem just got worse or if the lidocaine has caused the additional PVCs.

　　And what about lidocaine's effect on conduction velocity? Remember that conduction velocity is measured from the depth of the resting membrane (the most negative point of the cell's action potential) to the top of the action potential's slope (the most positive point). And remember that lidocaine decreases the resting membrane potential and raises the threshold potential. This means that lidocaine increases conduction velocity. Lidocaine can turn little flushes into big flushes.

　　This is one reason lidocaine is relatively contraindicated in atrial flutter and atrial fibrillation.[1,2] Say you have a patient in atrial fibrillation with a ventricular response of 100 per minute. If you administer lidocaine, the conduction velocity of those fibrillatory impulses may increase to the point that more of them conduct to the ventricles. Thus, the ventricular response may increase, cardiac output may decrease, and the patient's heart may become sicker.

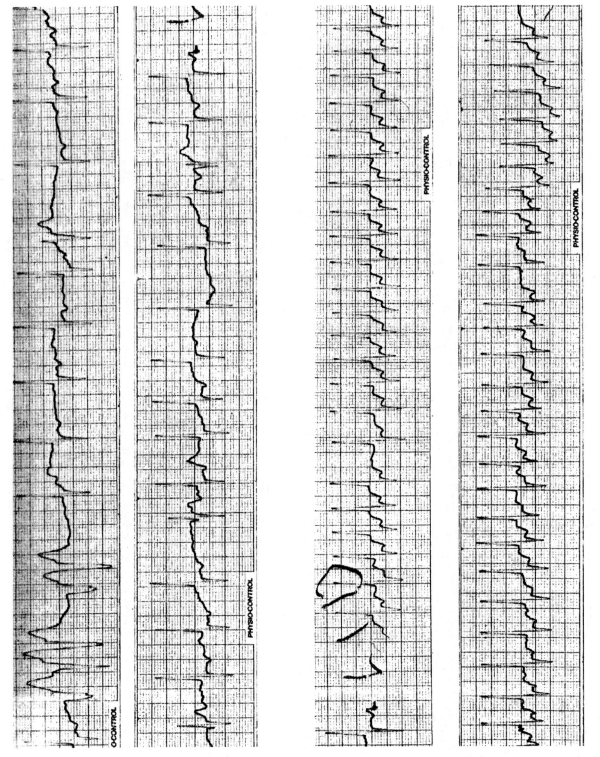

FIGURE 6.18

Take a look at Figure 6.18. This is a patient who was in atrial fibrillation, having what appeared to be PVCs. At the beginning of the top strip, you can see a run of these PVCs. The paramedic was especially concerned with these periods of ventricular tachycardia and administered lidocaine. The last two strips show you how the lidocaine affected this patient.

I can assure you that this patient's pain was not alleviated by the lidocaine administration. This patient's perfusion did not improve. This patient's anxiety level was not diminished. Thankfully, this patient did not progress into cardiac arrest. You can easily see, however, how lidocaine administration in the presence of atrial fibrillation may produce rapid ventricular responses that could cause ventricular fibrillation, cardiac arrest, or death.

SUMMARY

To acquire a basic understanding of electrophysiology is to gain a depth of understanding not usually offered to paramedics. If you carry this understanding into your clinical practice, you'll discover times when using it may, indeed, be life-saving for your patients.

REFERENCES

1. *Drug Facts and Comparisons*, J. B. Lippincott Co., St. Louis, MO, 1992; lidocaine, pp. 146f–h.
2. Marriott, H. J. and Bieza, C. F.: Alarming ventricular acceleration after lidocaine administration. *Chest* 1972, 61(7):682–3.

CHAPTER 7

Case Studies

Here is another chapter with a few case studies to help you review the things we've discussed in the previous chapters. As before, I'll be adding extra information as it occurs to me.

Figure 7.1 is the EKG of a 60-year-old gentleman who had a near-syncopal episode. He had vomited once (without blood in his emesis), denied chest pain, and was a little diaphoretic. His blood pressure was 120/60.

In leads II, III, and MCL_1 you can see sinus impulses, so he has a sinus tachycardia. He also has a normal axis. But he's got grouped beatings. And twice the shortest R-R interval is longer than the longest R-R interval. So what does that sound like? Right: type I A-V heart block (Wenckebach). The P-R intervals are supposed to change, but they don't. The P-R intervals actually stay the same, and they aren't very long. What's the usual pattern with a Wenckebach? Prolonged P-R interval that is conducted, more prolonged P-R interval that is conducted, and then a dropped (nonconducted) P wave. In Figure 7.1 the P-R interval is constant and within normal limits. Neither one of these points fits with our rules for type I A-V heart block, or Wenckebach. And where's the P wave that's supposed to be dropped?

It *is* a Wenckebach. But it's not an A-V Wenckebach. It's known as a sinus exit Wenckebach. The sinus node sits on the inside of the right atrium, near where the superior vena cava comes in. And it's not just one little point that fires—it is a section of tissue that generates impulses. What happens in a sinus exit Wenckebach is this: the impulse is formed and makes it out of the sinus node. The next one is formed and takes a little bit longer

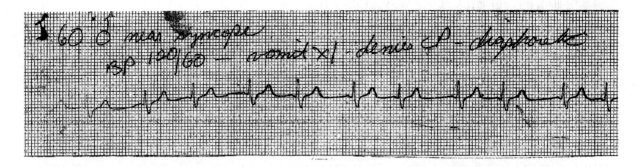

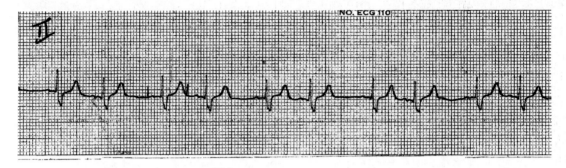

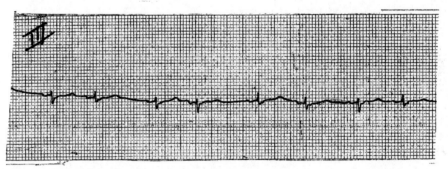

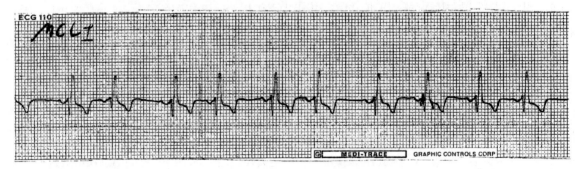

FIGURE 7.1

to exit the sinus node. And the next one is formed but doesn't make it out. It is blocked. The process then begins again. The difference here is that the P wave is reflective only of atrial conduction, not of sinus impulse formation. So, since we never see the sinus fire on the electrocardiogram, and the sinus fires *before* a P wave occurs, we don't see the blocked sinus impulse. The Wenckebach ventricular pattern is the same, but since the block is occurring in the sinus node, this is a little bit different. You can actually have Wenckebach-type behavior *anywhere* in the heart.

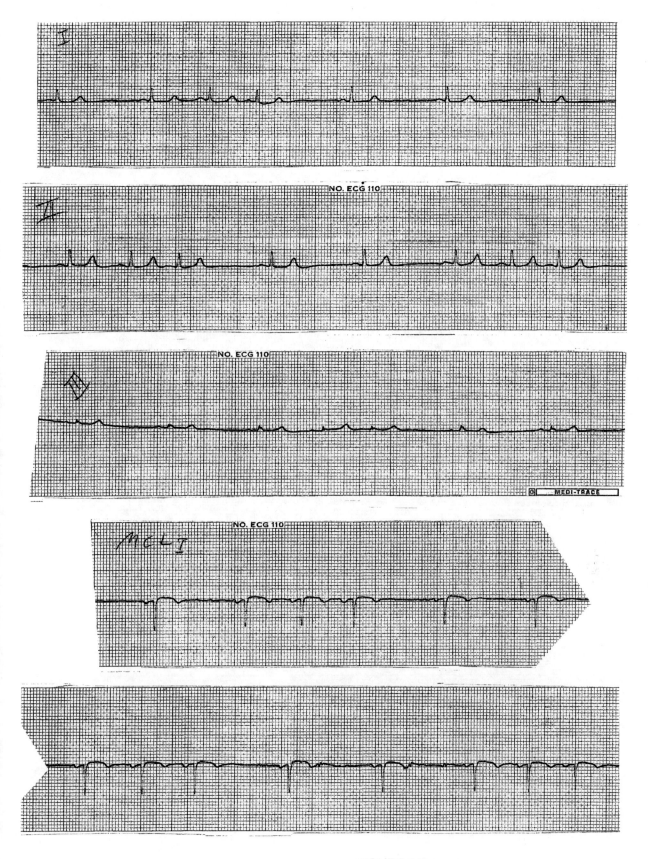

FIGURE 7.2

Figure 7.2 is another sinus exit Wenckebach. This is to show that these types of strips are not that uncommon—I cared for both of these patients (Syd complains that I got *all* the "good" cardiac patients). In Figure 7.2, however, you'll notice that the grouped beatings are irregular. The conduction ratio changes from 4:3 to 2:1 and back. This illustrates that Wenckebachs do not necessarily occur in fixed groups. Where the conduction ratio is 4:3, the R-R interval clearly shortens, and twice the shortest R-R interval is longer than the longest R-R interval (the one containing the blocked sinus impulse).

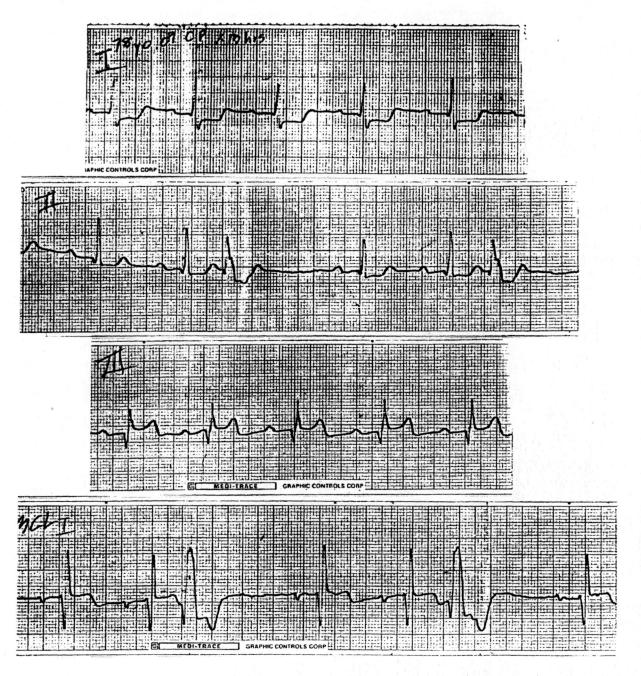

FIGURE 7.3

Figure 7.3 is the EKG of a 78-year-old male who had been having chest pain for 15 hours. He "just couldn't take it any more," so he finally called 911. We arrived to find him normotensive, with a respiratory rate of 24 and rales in both bases of his lungs. He was alert and well oriented, but (understandably) somewhat anxious. What do you think about his electrocardiogram?

Okay. He's got a sinus bradycardia (a rate of 52 to 56) with a normal axis—no hemiblocks. His P-R interval should catch your attention quickly. It's quite prolonged, about 0.28 seconds. Although you might not notice it in leads I or II, in leads III and MCL_1 you can see that his QRS complex measures about 0.14 seconds. MCL_1 shows that he has a right bundle branch block. His underlying rhythm is regular, but interrupted by unifocal PVCs in occasional trigeminy, which produces an even slower rate than that of 52 to 56.

While we looked at his EKG, the patient began to produce volumes of frothy, white sputum.

How do you mechanically treat fulminating pulmonary edema? With positive end-expiratory pressure (PEEP), after endotracheal intubation.* If you don't carry equipment specifically designed to provide positive end-expiratory pressure, you can use a Bag–Valve ventilation device to provide PEEP. Watch your intubated patient's breathing pattern as you assist the patient's natural inspiratory effort with Bag–Valve ventilation. When the patient exhales, gently squeeze the Bag–Valve device *against their exhalation.* This will create an increased amount of pressure in their lungs during expiration and assist in forcing the fluid of pulmonary edema back across the membranes. PEEP allows you to more effectively oxygenate and ventilate your patient.

Because he was awake, this patient required nasal intubation. Before nasally intubating a patient, it helps to prep the nose with Neo-Synephrine and a lubricant. But which patients present a contraindication to Neo-Synephrine? *Hypertensive* patients. Neo-Synephrine is a pure alpha-adrenergic drug that produces local vasoconstriction and may systemically affect the patient by increasing blood pressure.[1] Pulmonary edema is often associated with acute hypertension. If you have someone with a blood pressure of 220/140, you don't want to increase that, even a little, by squirting Neo-Synephrine in their nostrils. So *consider* NeoSynephrine—but only lubricate the nostrils in cases of hypertension.

What about lidocaine jelly? It lubricates and acts as a local anesthetic, diminishing some of the discomfort of passing a tube. Some physicians complain that lidocaine jelly dries the mucosa, causing nosebleeds later. We do need some kind of lubricant to pass the tube, however. And any water-soluble lubricant will do.

Once the nostrils (and tube) are lubricated, how do you nasally intubate an alert, agitated patient? You use bilateral soft wrist restraints. If you don't restrain the patient's hands, he will pull out the tube. And patients

---

*PEEP cannot be done with an oral airway and a bag-valve-mask. I've tried it. It doesn't work.

rarely remember to deflate the cuff prior to self-extubation! Restrain both wrists, keep him sitting bolt upright (even leaning slightly forward) and "talk him through the tube." Explain everything you are doing, as you are doing it. Take it slow, cue him to continue breathing, and nasally intubate him.

After intubation and with PEEP-assisted ventilation in progress, treat the causes of this patient's pulmonary edema: the bradycardia and PVCs. Lidocaine is definitely contraindicated in this gentleman. Not only does he have two blocks (prolonged P-R interval and right bundle branch block), but his bradycardia may be the cause of his PVCs. So gently administered atropine is in order.

Atropine can do several different things. It can produce ventricular tachycardia when someone has ventricular ectopy. But when someone has a rate this slow *and* ventricular ectopy, the atropine can increase the underlying rate and wipe out the ectopy. Also, when you increase cardiac output (by gently increasing the rate), you increase the emptying of the lungs by providing improved circulation for vascular diuresis.

With this particular patient, atropine increased his rate, wiped out his PVCs, and reversed his pulmonary edema (with the assistance of PEEP).

Let's take a look at Figure 7.4. This is the EKG of a 69-year-old male named Donald, "But call me Don." We found Don with right-sided hemiparesis, but able to talk, complaining of "a little bit of a headache." His skin color wasn't too bad, perhaps a little pale. He had a history of "a little bit of" hypertension, but wasn't on any medications. Don was indeed "a little bit" hypertensive (160/100). He had a heart rate as you see it, and a respiratory rate of 16.

Don has an underlying sinus rhythm. What is his axis? He has a pathologic left axis deviation (LAD), which indicates a left anterior hemiblock. He even demonstrates a little q wave in lead I and a little r wave in lead III, so his left anterior hemiblock is confirmed. He has a wide QRS complex. Looking at Don's MCL$_1$ strip, what bundle branch is blocked? He has a right bundle branch block. And he has multifocal PVCs. If you put it all together, the description of Don's EKG would sound like this: sinus rhythm, left axis deviation (thus left anterior hemiblock), right bundle branch block, with multifocal PVCs.

Would you like to medicate Don's multifocal PVCs with lidocaine? Absolutely not. His left anterior hemiblock combined with his right bundle branch block presents a precursor to complete heart block. Thus, Don's EKG provides evidence of a contraindication to lidocaine administration. Not to "whip a dead horse," but if you only looked at lead II, would you find the contraindication to lidocaine administration? Think about it. Probably not.

Here's another question: Do you have a desire to treat ventricular ectopy associated with what is probably a CVA? I'd be more inclined to treat the CVA. Certainly, you should be concerned about the multifocal PVCs. So how do you treat these PVCs? High-flow oxygen! That's always a good idea when your patient is having neurological deficits or ventricular ectopy.

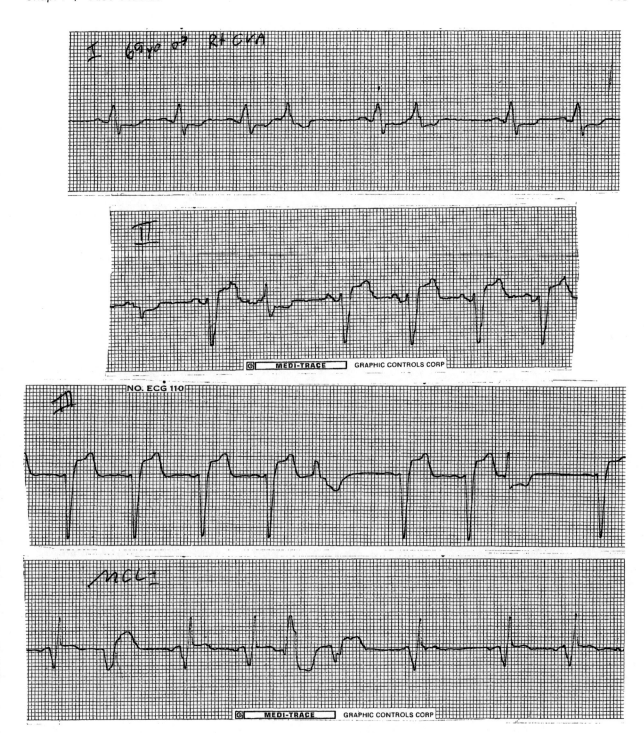

FIGURE 7.4

What about D_{50}? Hypoglycemia sometimes presents with hemiparesis, paleness, and diaphoresis. Where does the paleness and diaphoresis come from? It's from an adrenaline response, a sympathetic discharge. This same sympathetic discharge can also cause ventricular ectopy. So you actually may be able to treat Don's ventricular ectopy with dextrose.

Giving D_{50} to CVA patients opens up another can of worms, however. Recent literature suggests an adverse increase in brain infarct associated with the administration of 50% dextrose.[2,3] With that in mind, the best course of action would be to check the patient's blood sugar. If the patient's blood sugar is within normal limits, do not administer the dextrose.

If you don't have a reliable method of determining blood sugar content, then you need to administer a slow, *diluted* push of D_{50}. Access a vein with a large-bore angiocath, run the normal saline wide open, and then push the dextrose *without* crimping off the line. Observe the drip chamber. As you begin to administer the dextrose, the drip rate will diminish. Push the dextrose in slowly, maintaining the drip rate at TKO. As long as the IV fluid is still dripping, it means the dextrose is not backing up in the administration tubing. If it stops dripping, slow your pushing until the IV fluid resumes dripping. After the dextrose has been administered, reset the IV drip rate to TKO. In this way, you provide a slow, diluted dextrose administration that is kinder both to the patient's veins and to the patient.

Some people who answer your radio call for notification might not understand that a right bundle branch block with a left anterior hemiblock constitutes a contraindication to lidocaine administration. They might order you to give the lidocaine. How are you going to explain that you're *not* interested in giving lidocaine to this patient with multifocal PVCs? You can only use your best judgment. Perhaps you can insist on "deferral of lidocaine administration until the increased oxygenation has an opportunity to have an effect." If you are unable to defer the lidocaine administration, at the very least, you will administer it very slow push and be prepared for the patient to go into complete heart block.

REFERENCES

1. *Drug Facts and Comparisons*, J. B. Lippincott Co., St. Louis, MO, 1989: Neo-Synephrine, pp. 184–184d.

2. Browning, R. G.; Olson, D. W.; Stueven, H. A.; and Mateer, J. R.: 50% dextrose: antidote or toxin? *Ann Emerg Med* 1990,19(6):683–7.

3. Sieber, F. E. and Traystman, R. J.: Special issues: glucose and the brain. *Crit Care Med* 1992; 20 (1): 104–14.

CHAPTER **8**

Strategies for Diagnosis of Wide Complex Tachycardia

Welcome to Chapter Eight. Here, we'll be dealing with the arrhythmia that probably argues best and most emphatically for reading multiple-lead pre-hospital EKGs. Wide complex tachycardia is commonly misdiagnosed and mistreated. The mistreatment sometimes results in the patient's untimely death. Well, that's what we're here to avoid.

Wide complex tachycardia can be of supraventricular or ventricular origin. If ventricular in origin, the width of the QRS complex is due to the slower, retrograde activation of the myocardium. If supraventricular in origin, the width of the QRS complex is due to aberrant conduction through the ventricles.

Aberrant conduction is defined as a condition in which the cardiac electrical stimulus travels an abnormal, deviated pathway through the myocardium. This phenomenon can produce either an abnormally short P-R interval (such as pre-excitation syndromes) and/or an abnormally wide QRS complex.

An EKG similar to that of Figure 8.1 was once shown to over 196 practicing physicians (including several cardiologists).[1] A portion of this group considered their patient's vital signs while assessing the electrocardiogram. When they did so, 96 percent of these physicians and cardiologists made the wrong diagnosis. Consequently, they prescribed the wrong treatment. This EKG was also shown to 2500 practicing critical care unit nurses.[2] They did a bit better. Only 78 percent of them made the wrong diagnosis and prescribed the wrong treatment. At the end of the chapter we'll look at this EKG again. At that time, I promise you, with or without consideration of vital sign information, you will be able to make a correct diagnosis of this strip.

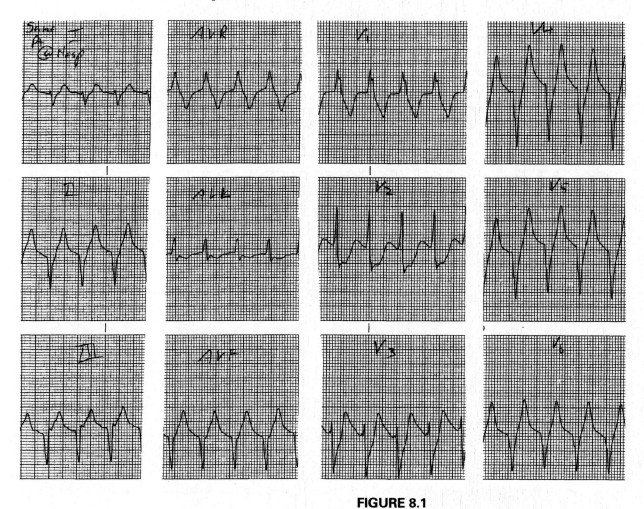

FIGURE 8.1

Figure 8.2 is the EKG of a patient who walked into the emergency room complaining of a "fluttering" in his chest. The patient was alert, had a blood pressure of 100/60, and had this wide complex tachycardia. When they saw his EKG, the emergency department team considered his blood pressure (over 100 systolic) and decided that this must be supraventricular tachycardia with aberrant ventricular conduction. So they gave him 5 mg of Verapamil. That was ineffective, so they gave him 10 mg more. That dropped his blood pressure a little bit, but didn't convert his rhythm. So they thought, "Oh gosh, maybe we made a mistake. Maybe this patient is in V tach!"

At that point they started giving him lidocaine. They gave him lidocaine until he got a little numb around his lips, and it didn't change anything. "Well, maybe we should go to Bretylium." So they gave him a loading dose of Bretylium. He vomited the way anyone does who gets Bretylium

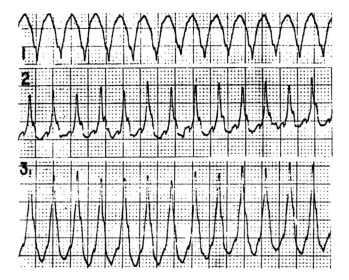

FIGURE 8.2 (Henry J. L. Marriott: *Practical Electrocardiography*, 8th ed., 1988; Williams & Wilkins, Baltimore.)

while conscious: copiously and with vigor. The Bretylium also dramatically dropped his blood pressure. But his rhythm still didn't convert. Now the ED staff had a hypotensive patient with a diminished level of consciousness, who was still in a wide complex tachycardia.

The next plan of attack was to get more "assertive." They cardioverted the patient at 50 watt-seconds, with no change in his rhythm. They tried again at 100 watt-seconds. Didn't work. They doubled *that* wattage, and it didn't work; 360 watt-seconds, no conversion. They did 30 consecutive cardioversions at 360 watt-seconds before one of the nurses happened to change the EKG lead. It was then that they identified the spikes of the patient's runaway artificial implanted pacemaker (Figure 8.3).

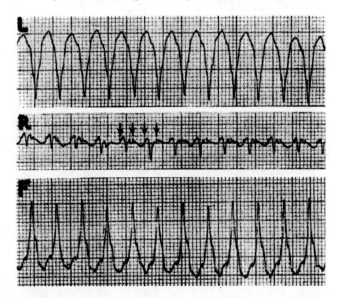

FIGURE 8.3 (Henry J. L. Marriott: *Practical Electrocardiography*, 8th ed., 1988; Williams & Wilkins, Baltimore.)

This patient died. Pacemakers are impressively resilient devices. You can squirt lidocaine all over them, it doesn't affect them in the least. Electricity doesn't bother them; they're built to survive numerous electrocutions. But the treatment for this patient would have been dramatically different had the patient's EKG been assessed accurately initially. In order to make an accurate assessment of any electrocardiogram, you must look in more than one lead. You must also have an idea of what you are looking for.

When confronted by somebody who is in a wide complex tachycardia, it is important to remember that ventricular tachycardia (and/or ventricular ectopy) is *more common* than supraventricular rhythms with aberrant ventricular conduction. If you apply all the criteria discussed in this chapter and you are still undecided whether a rhythm is ventricular tachycardia (V tach) or supraventricular tachycardia (SVT) with aberrant conduction, you are better off diagnosing and treating it as V tach. V tach is not only statistically more common, it is also more lethal.

Ventricular tachycardia (and/or ventricular ectopy) is *more common* than supraventricular rhythms with aberrant ventricular conduction.

Since most of us run leads I, II, and III first, let's begin with a brief review of axis. For differential diagnosis of V tach versus SVT with aberration, the only helpful axis is right shoulder axis. If you look at leads I, II, and III and the QRS complex deflections are all primarily negative, this means that the axis is pointing toward the right shoulder. Because right shoulder axis indicates retrograde impulse conduction throughout all the limb leads, this certainly favors V tach. Any other axis deviation is unhelpful, since it could be produced by either V tach or SVT.

Limb leads can also assist you with determining the width of the QRS complexes. QRS complexes wider than 0.14 seconds tend to favor ventricular ectopy or V tach. This is not a hard and fast rule, and there are no strong percentages to support this. But if the QRS complex is 0.14 seconds wide or wider, this *tends* to favor a ventricular rhythm.

Since limb leads provide little assistance when differentiating between V tach and SVT, you should quickly run through them and get to a lead that will give you the richest information. MCL_1 (or V_1) is the "gold mine lead." As with identifying bundle branch blocks, morphology of the QRS complexes in MCL_1 can help you identify V tach versus SVT with aberration.

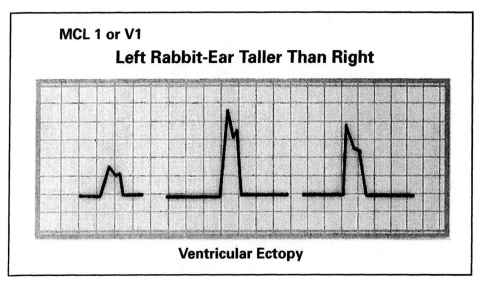

FIGURE 8.4

Figure 8.4 shows one of several MCL_1 QRS complex morphologies that favor V tach. If you have a patient with upright QRS complexes and there is a notch in the R waves, you have a QRS complex with "rabbit ears."

One day, years ago, a couple of nurses working in the coronary care unit at St. Anthony's Hospital in St. Petersburg, Florida, took Dr. Henry Marriott to lunch. They said, "We've been looking at 'rabbit ears.' And we think that, when the left rabbit ear is taller than the right rabbit ear, it indicates that the rhythm is ventricular in origin." Later research confirmed their hypothesis. If you observe a left rabbit ear taller than the right, this finding is highly indicative of ectopy.[3,4] In my opinion, this finding represents a 95 percent chance that the rhythm is ventricular tachycardia.

When using morphology to differentiate between supraventricular versus ventricular tachycardia, what you end up doing is "playing the percentages." If you observe a morphology that has a 90 percent chance (or better) of being one thing rather than another, those are pretty darn good odds—enough for a high comfort level when treating it. If, however, you observe a morphology with a poor percentage of accuracy, you need to seek other clues to make a differential diagnosis.

Back to rabbit ears. Rabbit ears don't have to be clearly "notched." Even a "slur" in the R wave can be considered a rabbit ear, and if the left side of the slur is taller than the right, there is still a 95 percent chance that the rhythm is V tach.

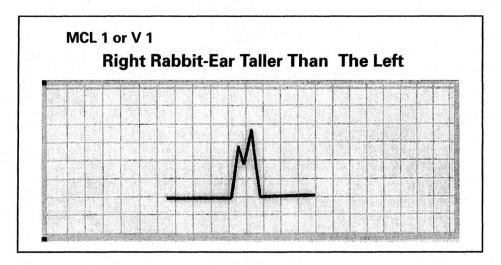

FIGURE 8.5

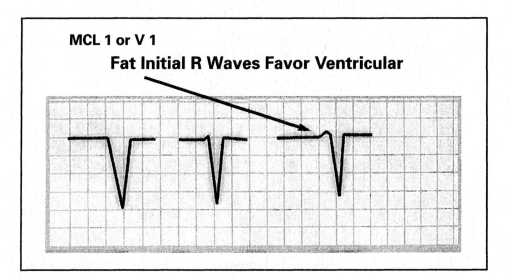

FIGURE 8.6

Some people make the mistake of thinking, "Hey. If a left rabbit ear taller than the right supports V tach, then a right rabbit ear taller than the left must support SVT." This is not at all true. If you have a right rabbit ear taller than the left (Figure 8.5) you have unusable information. If the right rabbit ear is taller than the left, there is not a high enough percentage to support a differential diagnosis for either V tach or SVT.

If you see a negative QRS complex in MCL_1 (V_1), like that of Figure 8.6, which bundle branch block is this morphology commonly associated with? Left bundle branch block. When a left bundle branch block is present, most patients have a predominantly negative QRS complex. Thirty percent of these patients have a thin, narrow r wave before a deep, wide QRS complex. But if you look at MCL_1 and see a negative QRS complex with a *fat* initial r wave (0.03 to 0.04 seconds wide or wider), there's a 90 percent chance that the rhythm is V tach. This percentage is sufficiently high enough to support a diagnosis of ventricular tachycardia.

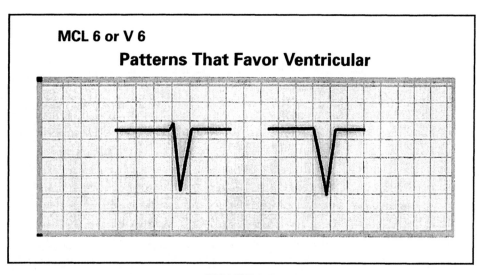

FIGURE 8.7

The next lead to look at when doing differential diagnosing between V tach and SVT with aberration is MCL_6 (V_6).

In MCL_6, if you see a completely negative QS complex (Figure 8.7), there is a 95 percent chance you're dealing with a ventricular rhythm. If you see a little r wave preceding a deep, wide S wave, there is an 87 percent chance that you're looking at a ventricular rhythm.

Another useful thing to assess is *precordial concordance.* Concordance is defined as an agreement or harmony between two (or more) factors. In electrocardiography, concordance is an agreement between the primary direction of QRS complex deflection in the precordial leads, V_1 through V_6.

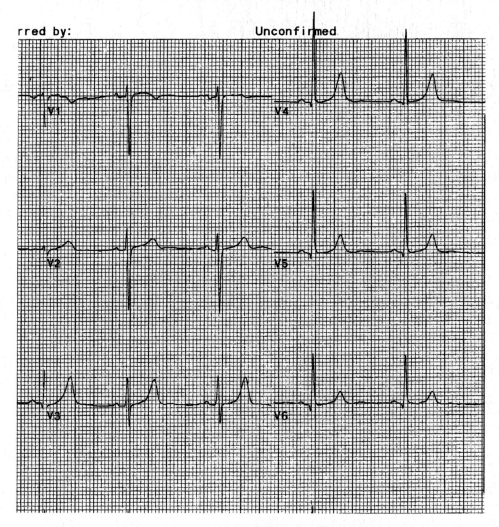

FIGURE 8.8

Figure 8.8 demonstrates the normal progression of QRS complex deflection through the V leads. As you can see, V_1 is usually negative and V_6 positive. Normally, there is a *lack* of precordial concordance.

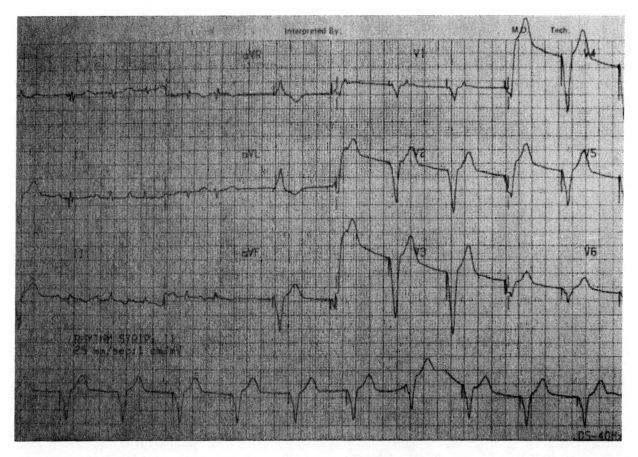

FIGURE 8.9

In Figure 8.9, however, you can see that the QRS complex deflection is negative throughout the V leads. Because of this, the V leads are referred to as having *negative precordial concordance,* or simply "negative concordance." Negative concordance is a powerful indicator that a rhythm has been generated in the ventricles—95 to 96 percent strong. This particular figure is easy to confirm as being ventricular, because you can see the spikes of the right ventricular transvenous pacemaker.

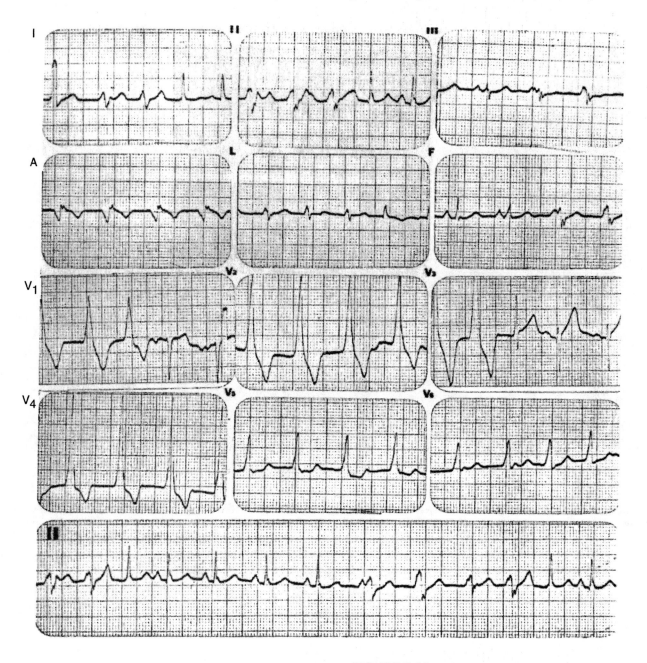

FIGURE 8.10

Positive concordance is precisely the opposite: all the QRS complex deflections in the V leads are upright, or positive. The presence of positive concordance is unusable information unless you can rule out Wolff–Parkinson–White (WPW) type A—a form of supraventricular pre-excitation. Positive concordance indicates either left ventricular tachycardia *or* SVT with WPW type A. Figure 8.10 is that of a V tach with positive concordance.

To observe for the absence or presence of V lead concordance in the field, run a strip of MCL_1 and then one of MCL_6. If they have opposite QRS complex deflections, there is an absence of concordance. If they each have positive QRS complex deflections, all the leads between would also contain upright QRS complexes. This is positive concordance. If both MCL_1 and MCL_6 have negative deflections, all the leads between would also have a negative deflection. This is negative concordance.

To sum-up concordance: Negative concordance strongly indicates ventricular tachycardia. Positive or absence of concordance can be either V tach or supraventricular tachycardia with aberration. And just because there is a normal progression of QRS complex directional changes through the V leads does *not* mean the rhythm is supraventricular. The only truly helpful concordance clue is negative concordance.

Concordance

- Negative concordance strongly indicates ventricular tachycardia.
- Positive concordance can be either V tach or supraventricular tachycardia with aberration.
- Absence of concordance (a normal progression of QRS complex directional changes through the V leads) does *not* mean the rhythm is supraventricular.
- The only truly helpful concordance clue is negative concordance.

What about morphologies that favor SVT with aberration?

A triphasic complex in MCL_1—a QRS complex that goes above the baseline, below the baseline, and back above the baseline—has a 90 percent chance of being SVT with aberration, and not ventricular tachycardia. You should recognize this complex (Figure 8.11) as being the R-S-R prime (RSR') morphology of a right bundle branch block.

A triphasic complex in MCL_6 (small q wave, an R wave, and an S wave) also has a 90 percent chance of being SVT with aberration. It is probably not ventricular tachycardia.

What about heart rates? On the first day of your first EKG class, you were probably taught about heart rate being one factor in the process of interpreting a heart rhythm. When dealing with wide beat tachycardias, however, the rate is only diagnostically significant when it climbs above 250 per minute.

Let's review idioventricular rates. Idioventricular rhythms are supposed to range between a rate of 20 to 40 beats per minute. Accelerated idioventricular rhythms range from 40 to 100 beats per minute. And ventricular tachycardia can range from 100 to 250.

What about junctional rhythms? The inherent rate is supposed to be 40 to 60 beats per minute. Yet we've seen junctional bradycardias as slow as, say, 30 beats per minute. Accelerated junctional rhythms range from 60 to 100 beats per minute, and junctional tachycardias from 100 to maybe 250.

The rate of a normal sinus rhythm is supposed to be between 60 and 100. Sinus bradycardias may get as slow as 30 beats per minute. Sinus tachycardias can range from 100 to 150. And atrial tachycardias may fire as fast as 250.

If we put all this together, it looks like this:

- Idioventricular rhythms can range from 30 to 250.
- Junctional rhythms can range from 30 to 250.
- Sinus or atrial rhythms can range from 30 to 250.

Until you are dealing with a heart rate above 250 beats per minute, rate is of little help in differentiating origins of rhythms. Once you get up around the 300 mark, however, it is highly unlikely that the ventricles are generating the rhythm.

What about regularity versus irregularity? Is this a criterion for differentiating supraventricular rhythms with aberration and ventricular rhythms? Yes and no.

Aberrantly conducted supraventricular rhythms can be regular or irregular. So can ventricular rhythms. Ventricular tachycardia can be very irregular when it's starting or stopping. The only potential differentiating factor is that, once V tach has taken hold, it tends to be very regular. It's usually only irregular when starting or stopping.

Atrial or junctional tachycardias tend to be the same way. They may be irregular when starting or stopping, but when they are fully involved, they are very regular.

So when you're looking at a wide beat tachycardia that is regular, it's either supraventricular tachycardia with aberrancy or ventricular tachycardia.

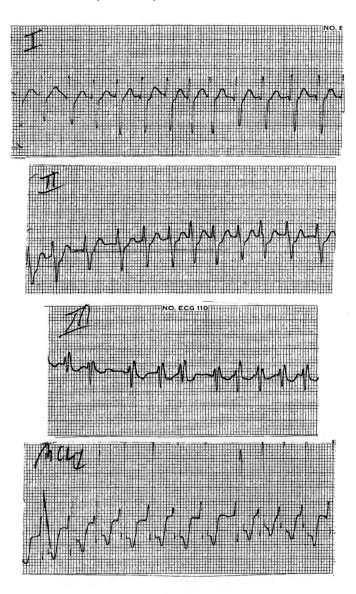

FIGURE 8.11

But when you're looking at a wide beat tachycardia that *persists* as being irregularly irregular, you're probably looking at a supraventricular rhythm with aberrancy (atrial fibrillation or atrial flutter with varying ventricular response).

In the preceding paragraphs, I've presented a plethora of clues to use when you need to differentiate V tach from SVT with aberration. Right about now you may be asking yourself, "How do I put all this together so that I can *use* it?"

There is a landmark study that was published in the May 1991 edition of *Circulation* that I think is probably one of the most important recently published papers on differential diagnosis of wide complex tachycardia.[5] The authors of this study looked at 554 wide complex tachycardias. Of these, 384 were found to be ventricular tachycardia, and 170 were supraventricular tachycardia with aberration. That's a pretty good representation of the normal ratio. As I mentioned earlier, in wide complex tachycardias, ventricular tachycardia is more common.

This research study had a very high sensitivity and specificity ratio. For those of you who aren't "into" research, this means that the project was set up well and obtained results that can be considered valid. The authors developed an algorithm for differential diagnosis of V tach versus SVT with aberration. To use their strategy to its fullest potential, a 12-lead electrocardiogram is required. However, their algorithm is just as useful for those of us who run leads I, II, III, MCL$_1$, and MCL$_6$ in the field.

Step 1: Look across the precordial leads (V$_1$ through V$_6$, or MCL$_1$ and MCL$_6$). If they all contain negative QS complexes, then you've got V tach. And, using their system of steps, once you see negative concordance, you don't need to look at anything else on the EKG. You can initiate treatment for V tach with a high level of confidence that you're approaching things correctly. If negative concordance is not present, you move to step 2.

Step 2: Measure the R-S interval in all the precordial leads with clear R and S waves. Basically, the R-S interval is measured from the beginning of the QRS complex to the initial *point* of the S wave—the point of the first negative impulse after the R wave. Is it less or greater than 0.10 seconds (100 milliseconds)? If the R-S interval is greater than 0.10 seconds, you have V tach, and you don't need to look at anything else. You can initiate treatment for V tach, confident that you're approaching things correctly. If the R-S interval is less than 0.10 seconds (2.5 little boxes), you move to step 3.

Step 3: Look for A-V dissociation. Now, remember that people with "P preoccupation syndrome" can find P waves on an electroencephalogram (see the footnote in Chapter One). For the rest of us, however, it is sometimes very difficult to find P waves in a wide complex tachycardia electrocardiogram. If you *can* find P waves and they are dissociated from the QRS complexes, you are dealing with ventricular tachycardia. You may stop looking for clues and treat the V tach. If you can't find P waves or can't tell whether they are clearly dissociated or not, move to step 4.

Step 4: This is based on observation of the same morphologic clues that we've previously discussed. In MCL$_1$ (V$_1$), look for a left rabbit ear taller than the right. Or, if MCL$_1$ is a negative complex, look for a fat initial R wave followed by a deep, wide S. If MCL$_1$ isn't helpful, go to MCL$_6$ (V$_6$) and look for a QS complex. If that morphology isn't present, is there a little r wave before a deep, wide S wave in MCL$_6$? Any of these findings identify the rhythm as ventricular tachycardia.

If you've gone through all these steps and not found an indication for V tach, then the rhythm is SVT with aberration.

The reason I find this algorithm so spectacular is that it sets you up to find V tach *first*. V tach is considerably more lethal than SVT with aberration, occurs more often, and is more commonly mistreated. I'm presenting this algorithm here, and also including it in the appendix.

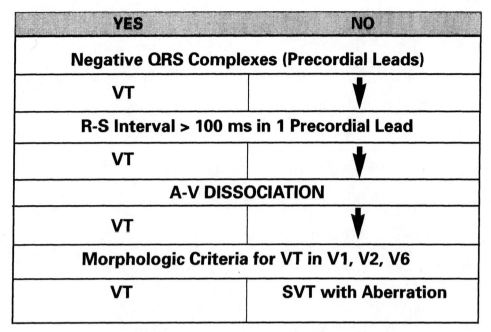

YES	NO
Negative QRS Complexes (Precordial Leads)	
VT	▼
R-S Interval > 100 ms in 1 Precordial Lead	
VT	▼
A-V DISSOCIATION	
VT	▼
Morphologic Criteria for VT in V1, V2, V6	
VT	**SVT with Aberration**

Algorithm for differentiating V tach from SVT with aberration.

Let's walk through a couple of examples.

Figure 8.12 is a 12-lead EKG. If you're not running 12 leads in the field, just look at leads I, II, III, V_1, and V_6. Actually, for the differential diagnosis of a wide beat tachycardia, those are the primary leads we're going to look at on a 12 lead anyway.

Although determining axis is not part of the *Circulation* authors' algorithm, I prefer to include it. You can consider it to be step A, if you like. Look at leads I, II, and III to determine the axis. There is a negative complex in I, a negative complex in II, and a negative complex in III. This is a right shoulder axis, also known as "No Man's Land" axis. Right shoulder axis is highly indicative of V tach. So this is a big clue in favor of V tach.

Now let's begin with the first step of the algorithm, by looking across the V leads. V_1 is primarily positive, and V_6 is primarily negative. There is an absence of concordance. Specifically, there is an absence of negative concordance. So, finding no helpful information, we move to the next step.

Measure the precordial R-S interval. Since the R-S interval in Figure 8.12 is greater than 0.10 seconds in at least one precordial lead, we can stop at this point. With this finding, the EKG has told us enough to be able to treat this patient for V tach! For the sake of practice, however, we will continue through the algorithm.

Next, is there A-V dissociation? In this electrocardiogram, it is difficult to identify atrial activity. And if you have a hard time finding atrial activity, it's very difficult to decide whether or not there is AV dissociation.

Step 4 is to look for specific morphological clues in V_1. Looking at V_1, you see a left rabbit ear taller than the right. With this finding alone, there is a 95 percent chance that this patient is in ventricular tachycardia. With this finding, we could stop and treat the patient for V tach.

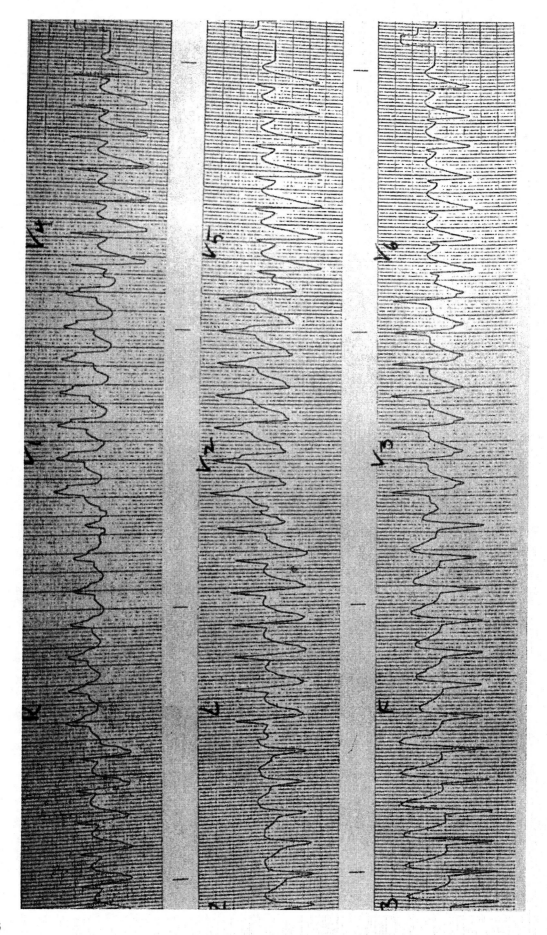

FIGURE 8.12

136

Since we're continuing on for practice, look at V_6. You can see a little R wave and a deep, wide S wave. These indicate an 87 percent chance of V tach. Again, we could stop and treat this patient for V tach.

This particular EKG (Figure 8.12) has a multitude of strong differential diagnostic clues. The right shoulder axis was a pretty good clue even before using the algorithm. Step 1 was unhelpful, but step 2 (identifying a precordial R-S interval greater than 0.10 seconds) provided enough information to stop right there and treat the patient for ventricular tachycardia.

Had we needed to proceed to step 3, the absence of clear atrial activity (with which to determine presence of AV dissociation) would have prompted us to move to step 4. But step 4 contained two very strong morphological indications (in both V_1 and V_6) that the rhythm was V tach.

Let's discuss treatment for a moment. Let's say that the patient with the EKG in Figure 8.12 has a blood pressure of 150/100 and is alert and well oriented. But he is complaining of a "fluttering" sensation in his chest, some weakness, and a little nausea. How many of you were taught that you always treat your patient, not the patient's EKG? (Reader, raise your hand if you were taught that.) If this were the case 100 percent of the time, would you give this patient lidocaine or not? If you don't give him lidocaine, you'll be leaving him in V tach. What will happen to the patient if you leave him in V tach? He's certainly not likely to get better on his own. He needs the lidocaine. And we're going to give him lidocaine. So are we treating the EKG? No, we're not going to squirt lidocaine on the EKG. But we are going to give this patient lidocaine *despite* his adequate mentation and sufficient blood pressure, based solely upon his life-threatening arrhythmia.

V tach is the exception to the "treat the patient, not the EKG" rule. No matter how "good" the patient looks, how sufficient his blood pressure, how well he's mentating, V tach needs to be stopped before the patient goes into cardiac arrest. So please stop telling students to "treat the patient, not the EKG." Please teach students instead to treat the patient "in concert with the EKG." Or "treat the patient, not the EKG—except for V tach."

When you use this algorithm and find an indication for V tach, you treat the patient for V tach. If, however, you go through all the steps *without* finding an indication to treat the patient for V tach, you then treat the patient for supraventricular tachycardia with aberration. It's as simple as that.

But let's say we didn't trust our algorithm, and we incorrectly diagnosed a rhythm as V tach. Most of the time, treating SVT with aberration as V tach by giving lidocaine does not cause significant problems.[6] *Most* of the time. A certain percentage of SVT patients has a *fixed* bundle branch block, not transient aberration. For them, lidocaine may impair conduction through the A-V node. This can cause the patient to go from a tachycardia to complete heart block.

On the other hand, if patients in V tach are misdiagnosed as being in SVT with aberration, administration of Verapamil can *easily kill them.* I mention this to illustrate that it's safer to err on the side of V tach if you cannot make a differential diagnosis. Not only is V tach more common

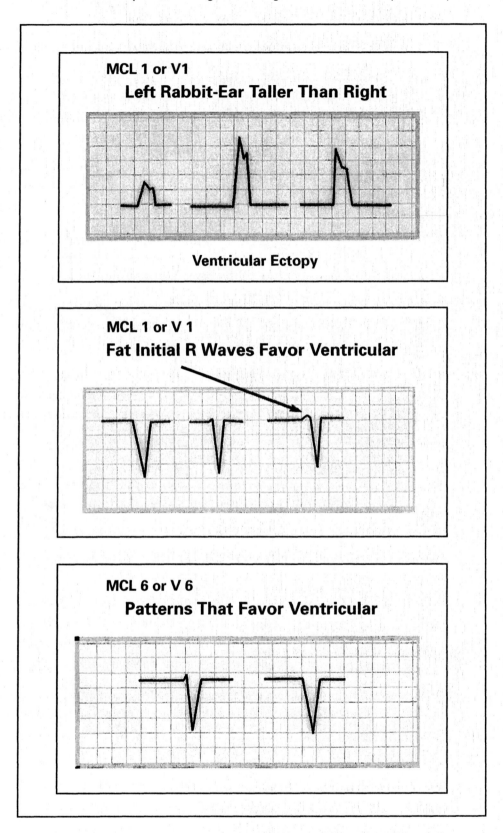

Morphological clues highly suggestive of V tach.

than SVT with aberration, but a patient in SVT has a better chance of surviving incorrect treatment.

If you can't clearly differentiate, but you strongly feel that the patient is in SVT with aberration, the safest choice for treating the SVT would be administration of adenosine (Adenocard). To date (and I stress "to date"), there have been no reported adverse occurrences when adenosine was administered to patients in V tach. Of course, it didn't convert the V tach. But receiving adenosine didn't kill them either.

One treatment choice that some people consider safe for V tach and SVT alike is cardioversion. "If you can't tell the difference, you can always electrocute them," they say…. Although electricity may be the bottom-line treatment for both, I'm uncomfortable with such a cavalier attitude.

I was in an emergency department one day when a 38-year-old male was brought in with a wide complex tachycardia. The attending physician called in a cardiologist to deal with it. The cardiologist who responded was 87-years-old. He had a stethoscope around his neck with tubes the size of garden hoses, supporting a gigantic bell, and he was walking with a cane. I approached him and asked, "Are you gonna cardiovert him?" If he was, I planned to call my dispatcher and see if we could stay out of service to watch the cardioversion. Well, the cardiologist looked at me, tilted his head, and said, "You're one of those paramedic guys, aren't you?"

"Yes. Yes, sir, I am."

And he replied, "I think paramedics are a good idea. We didn't have paramedics when I got started in medicine." He then proceeded to tell me his life history.

"You know, I've been practicing medicine for 54 years now. And right after medical school, I took an interest in the heart. They didn't call us cardiologists back then. But I've learned a lot of rules for cardiology over the years. And every single rule I've ever learned has either been thrown out or I've seen an exception to it. Except for one rule. And that rule is this: after you apply electricity to somebody's heart, the resulting rhythm is always the same, 100 percent of the time. Do you know what that rhythm is, son? Asystole. At least for a short period of time, electricity always produces asystole. When I was in medical school, asystole meant 'death.' And I don't think we should go around creating death. So, no son, as long as he can still talk to me, I'm not going to cardiovert that man."

I thought that was a pretty good testimonial to the use of cardioversion only after all else has failed.

So let's get back to our practice of using the algorithm for differential diagnosis of wide complex tachycardias.

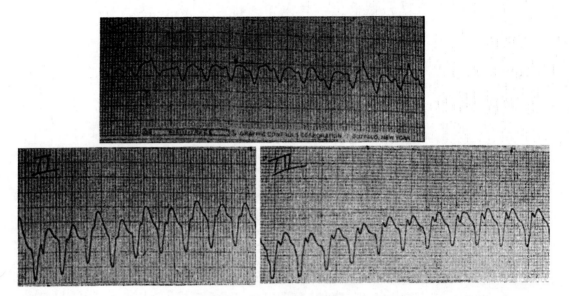

FIGURE 8.13

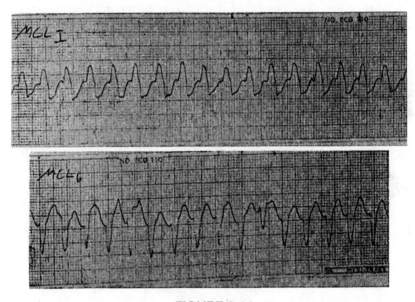

FIGURE 8.14

Looking at leads I, II, and III of Figure 8.13, you can see that this patient has a right shoulder axis. This immediately should increase your suspicion that the rhythm is V tach.

MCL_1 and MCL_6 have opposite primary directions of deflection, meaning there is an absence of concordance. This does not help you differentiate SVT from V tach.

Measure the R-S intervals of MCL_1 and MCL_6. You find that the R-S in MCL_1 is greater than 0.10 seconds. This EKG rhythm is V tach. You don't need to look for AV dissociation, and you don't need to look at the morphology of MCL_1 or MCL_6. You can stop right now and treat this patient for ventricular tachycardia.

Although you don't need to look for morphological clues in this EKG, let's review them for practice. Figure 8.14 is the MCL$_1$ and MCL$_6$ leads of Figure 8.13's patient.

Do you see the little bit of a slur on the R wave in MCL$_1$ in Figure 8.14? Remember that rabbit ears do not have to be notched. A slur is also considered a "rabbit ear." In this upright QRS complex, the left side of the slur is a little bit taller than the right side. Left rabbit ear taller than the right, *in MCL$_1$*, is V tach.

Let's say we wanted to check for morphological clues, but looked at MCL$_6$ before MCL$_1$. In this particular EKG, we still would have cause to immediately stop and treat for V tach. The MCL$_6$ in Figure 8.14 has a little r wave followed by a deep, wide S wave. This is V tach. Treat this patient now.

Figure 8.15 shows the MCL$_1$ lead of a patient with a run of funny looking beats. What does the underlying rhythm lok like? It's grossly irregular and there are no discernible P waves. Atrial fibrillation. In atrial fibrillation and atrial flutter, the rule about percentages in V tach versus SVT is reversed. In the majority of rhythms, ectopy is more common than aberration. In atrial fibrillation and atrial flutter, however, aberration is more common than ectopy.

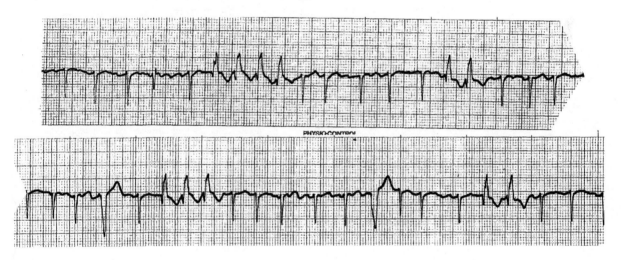

FIGURE 8.15

In atrial fibrillation and atrial flutter, aberration is more common than ectopy.

The EKG strip in Figure 8.15 introduces a new term and a new set of criteria. We've already established that the underlying rhythm is atrial fibrillation. Notice that the FLBs have an RSR' pattern. This is an example of right bundle branch block aberration. But why were those particular beats conducted aberrantly? Because those impulses penetrated the ventricles before the refractory period of the right ventricle was completed.

One rule of refractory periods is this: the time required for ventricular repolarization is established by the previous R-R interval. The longer the R-R interval is, the longer the refractory period required for the next repolarization. If an impulse arrives early, repolarization is incomplete, and aberrant conduction may occur. This is seen on the electrocardiogram as a long R-R followed by a premature complex (a shorter R-R) that is wide and bizarre.

The time required for ventricular repolarization is established by the duration of the previous R-R interval. An early impulse may create aberrant conduction.

When the underlying rhythm is atrial fibrillation, and a long R-R is followed by a short R-R, producing an aberrantly conducted QRS complex, it is called *Ashman's phenomenon*. Unless you were familiar with this phenomenon, you would probably consider these wide and bizarre complexes to be PVCs. If the premature impulse is repeated immediately, a pattern that mimics ventricular tachycardia may occur (Figure 8.16).

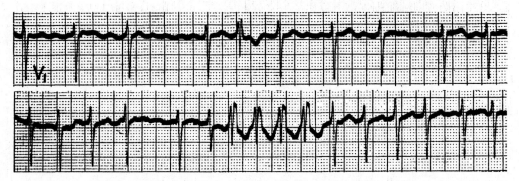

FIGURE 8.16 (Henry J. L. Marriott: *Practical Electrocardiography*, 8th ed., 1988; Williams & Wilkins, Baltimore.)

If you are quick enough to hit the record button and capture the first beat of the run when you see a burst of wide beat tachycardia *in MCL₁*, look closely at the first wide complex. Many times, only the first beat will have the RSR' morphology. Complexes that follow rapidly may lose the initial R wave because of the rapid rate.

An RSR' pattern in MCL₁ is the most frequent aberrant pattern to occur with Ashman's phenomenon. This is because the right bundle branch normally requires more time to repolarize than the left. Thus, a premature beat is more likely to find the right bundle branch "blocked" because of incomplete repolarization, and the RSR' morphology of right bundle branch block will be seen. However, any pattern of aberrant conduction is possible (Figure 8.17).

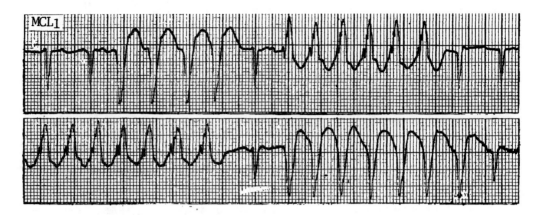

FIGURE 8.17 (Henry J. L. Marriott: *Practical Electrocardiography*, 8th ed., 1988; Williams & Wilkins, Baltimore.)

Ashman's phenomenon is a label that is only applied to atrial fibrillation with this sort of aberrancy. If it occurs with any other underlying rhythm, it is called a rate-dependent bundle branch block. Figures 8.18 and 8.19 show examples of rate-dependent bundle branch blocks.

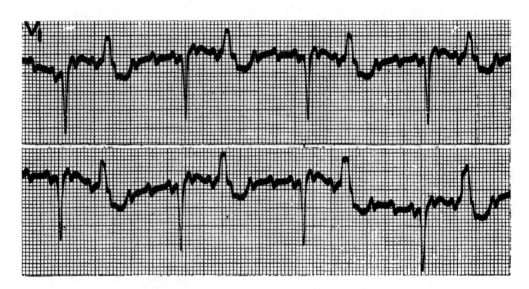

FIGURE 8.18 (Henry J. L. Marriott: *Practical Electrocardiography*, 8th ed., 1988; Williams & Wilkins, Baltimore.)

Figure 8.18 shows an atrial flutter with alternating 2:1 and 4:1 conduction. The shorter cycles (where the rate is more rapid) exhibit a right bundle branch block conduction aberration.

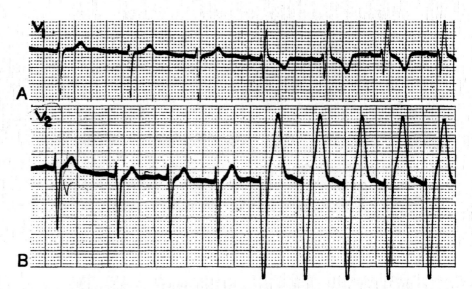

FIGURE 8.19 (Henry J. L. Marriott: *Practical Electrocardiography,* 8th ed., 1988; Williams & Wilkins, Baltimore.)

Strip A of Figure 8.19 is the sinus rhythm of a 19-year-old female whose rate has been increased by exercise. The faster rate causes a rate-dependent right bundle branch block to develop. Strip B is the sinus rhythm of a 64-year-old male with severe coronary disease. When his rate accelerates, he develops a rate-dependent left bundle branch block.

Okay. Say you didn't know about Ashman's phenomenon, and you thought the patient in Figure 8.15 was throwing PVCs. What would be the problem with giving lidocaine to this patient? This is something that's bothered me for years. None of the paramedic textbooks I've ever seen (and darn few of the cardiology textbooks) discuss the relative contraindication for lidocaine in atrial fibrillation or atrial flutter. This contraindication is especially true for atrial fibrillation with rapid ventricular response.

Lidocaine can accelerate the ventricular rate of patients in atrial fibrillation or flutter.[7] This is because lidocaine sometimes shortens AV node conduction time, allowing more atrial impulses to get through to the ventricles.[8] So you can take somebody with a heart rate around 150 (like Figure 8.15) and give them a heart rate of about 250 by administering lidocaine. Because of this, I would strongly discourage you from using lidocaine in the presence of atrial fib—especially when ventricular response is already rapid.

Our next case involves a 36-year-old gentleman with a chief complaint of sickle cell crisis, a genetic disease that primarily afflicts black people. Maurice has sickle cell anemia, and he knows when he's in crisis. Before we discuss his EKG, let's review the triad of treatment for sickle cell crisis.[9]

High-flow oxygen is the first treatment for sickle cell crisis because sickle-shaped red blood cells can no longer carry oxygen. Second is fluid administration. Aggressive hydration is required to compensate for the fluid losses from fever, vomiting, or diarrhea that frequently accompany sickle cell crisis. Hydration also helps to mitigate the sludging of sickled erythrocytes and flush the sickled cells through the capillaries. (An average adult in sickle cell crisis could reasonably be given 1 to 2 liters of fluid, depending upon local protocols.) Third, administer morphine. Vascular occlusion from sickle-shaped blood cells clumping together and obstructing blood flow to the tissues beyond is impressively painful. Morphine is good for both pain control and peripheral vascular dilation. This allows the sickled cells to pass through smaller vascular avenues, diminishing the areas of necrosis caused by sickle cell occlusion.

It's fortunate that, in this country, most people who have sickle cell anemia know they've got it. They also know the treatment. Unfortunately, many medical professionals are unfamiliar with the proper treatment. Thus, young black persons who insist that they need morphine may not receive proper treatment. Someone in sickle cell crisis needs plenty of oxygen, fluid, and morphine.

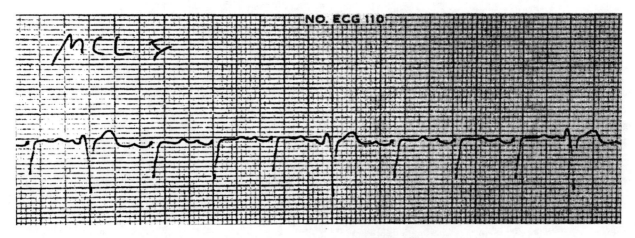

FIGURE 8.20

Looking at Maurice's EKG in Figure 8.20 (MCL_1 lead only), you can see some early QRS complexes. They are negative and have a fat initial r wave preceding a deep, wide S wave. Each has a P wave in front of it. When you look for P waves to determine the presence or absence of A-V dissociation (Step 3 of the algorithm), be very careful. Consider the timing and morphology of all the P waves seen. And carefully examine the P-R intervals. Maurice's early complexes are PVCs. They are referred to as *end diastolic PVCs*, because they each occur after a normally timed P wave.

Maurice was delivered to a teaching hospital's emergency room. His EKG was shown to no less than 13 physicians! All of them determined that the early complexes were PACs with aberration because of the P waves in front of them.

The term PAC means *premature atrial contraction*. There is nothing "P" about the "AC"s in this EKG. The P waves, if you "map them out," do not come early. They are right in time with all the others. And if these wide and bizarre QRS complexes were initiated by the timely P waves preceding them, it makes no sense at all for them to have a shorter P-R interval than that of the other PQRST complexes. In fact, most often, PACs will have longer P-R intervals than the underlying rhythm.

Consequently, the wide and bizarre complexes are PVCs. Maurice's PVCs just happen to fall immediately after normally timed atrial depolarizations. They are *end diastolic*, right ventricular PVCs.

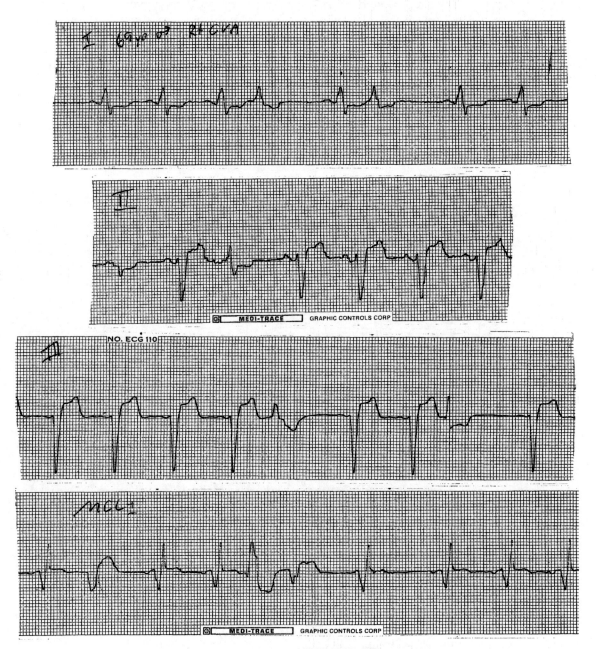

FIGURE 8.21

You may recognize Figure 8.21 as being the same as Figure 7.4. This is the EKG of a 69-year-old man named Don, who had right-sided hemiparesis. We previously determined that Don had an underlying sinus rhythm, a pathologic left axis deviation (indicating a left anterior hemiblock), and a right bundle branch block, with multifocal PVCs.

Take a look at the differing morphologies of QRS complexes in Don's MCL$_1$ strip. The first QRS complex shows his underlying rhythm and exhibits his right bundle branch block. We know he has a right bundle branch block because of the turn signal method.

Now take a look at the second complex in Don's MCL$_1$ lead. The MCL$_1$ electrode sits in the fourth intercostal space, just to the right of the patient's sternum. The second impulse is early, wide, and bizarre. Unlike Don's underlying rhythm this impulse is negative. This indicates that the impulse is going away from the MCL$_1$ electrode, which means that this impulse is a right ventricular PVC, a PVC that started in the right ventricle.

On the other hand, the fifth impulse in Don's MCL$_1$ is early, wide, and bizarre and has a left rabbit ear taller than the right. This is a left ventricular PVC. It's upright in MCL$_1$, so that means it is traveling toward the MCL$_1$ electrode. Thus, it originates in the left ventricle, the ventricle that is farther away from the MCL$_1$ electrode.

It would be a mistake to think that either of these patterns is generated from a supraventricular impulse with aberrant ventricular conduction, because Don already has a right bundle branch block. So you know what his aberrant ventricular pattern looks like. If anything changed because of a supraventricular early beat, it would result in a block of both ventricles, and you would see a nonconducted atrial premature beat.

The last figure of this chapter is a repeat of the first figure from this chapter. Let's see if you can do better than 96 percent of the physicians (including several cardiologists) and 78 percent of the critical care nurses who were unable to correctly diagnose this EKG.

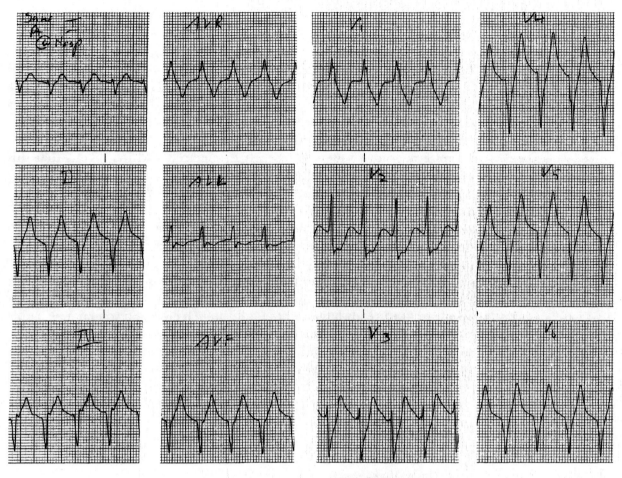

FIGURE 8.22

What is the axis of Figure 8.22? Right shoulder axis. We already find a high-percentage clue that this EKG is not SVT with aberration. Now let's apply the *Circulation* authors' algorithm for differentiating SVT from V tach.

There is no negative concordance, so that tells us nothing definitive. We move on.

The next step is to measure the R-S interval in those precordial leads that exhibit clear R and S waves (V_2 and V_3). Remember, the R-S interval is measured from the beginning of the QRS complex to the initial *point* of the S wave—the point of the first negative impulse after the R wave. Is the R-S interval in either of these leads greater than 0.10 seconds (100 milliseconds)? V_2 has an R-S of exactly 0.10 seconds. In V_3, if you count the first little "nub" as part of the R wave, the R-S measures 0.08 seconds. So let's move to step 3 of the *Circulation* authors' algorithm.

There are no consistently clear lumps, bumps, blips, or dips suggestive of atrial activity. Thus, we cannot determine the presence of A-V dissociation.

So now we need to look at morphological clues. Look at V_1. It clearly has a left rabbit ear taller than the right. There should no longer be any question in your mind that this is V tach. Next look at V_6. It has a little r wave followed by a deep wide S wave—again, indicative of V tach.

Looking at the overall strip, what is it? It's V tach.

SUMMARY

So how'd you do? Did you have trouble diagnosing this as V tach (like many cardiologists and CCU nurses)? If so, I'd encourage you to review this chapter until you feel more comfortable with it. This is one topic where your mastery of the material can make a difference between life and death.

REFERENCES

1. Morady, F.; Baerman, J. M.; DiCarlo, L. A.; et al., A prevalent misconception regarding wide-complex tachycardia. *JAMA* 1985; 254:2790–2792.

2. Cooper, J.; and Marriott, H. J. L.: Why are so many critical-care nurses unable to recognize ventricular tachycardia in the 12-lead electrocardiogram? *Heart Lung* 1989; 18: 243–247.

3. Gozensky, C.; and Thorne, D.: Rabbit ears: an aid in distinguishing ventricular ectopy from aberration. *Heart and Lung* 1974:3, 634.

4. Marriott, H. J.: Differential diagnosis of supraventricular and ventricular tachycardia. *Cardiology* 1990;77(3): 209–20.

5. Brugada, P.; Brugada, J.; Mont, L.; Smeets, J.; and Andries, E. W.: A new approach to the differential diagnosis of a regular tachycardia with a wide QRS complex. *Circulation* 1991; 83:1649–59.

6. Wrenn, K.: Management strategies in wide QRS complex tachycardia. *Am J Emerg Med* 1991; 9(6): 592–97.

7. Marriott, H. J.; and Bieza C.F.: Alarming ventricular acceleration after lidocaine administration. *Chest* 1972; 61(7): 682–3.

8. *Drug Facts and Comparisons*, J. B. Lippincott Co., St. Louis, MO: May 1992, lidocaine HCL, p. 146f.

9. Lee, G. R., et al.; *Wintrobe's Clinical Hematology*, 9th ed., 1993. Lea & Febiger, Philadelphia, pp 1062–85.

CHAPTER 9

Pre-excitation Syndromes

Pre-excitation syndromes occur when a supraventricular impulse activates part or all of the ventricles via an accessory path of conduction. Thus, the ventricles are activated earlier than they would have been had the impulse traveled via normally routed conduction. Normal conduction begins at the SA node and travels through the atria to the A-V node/junction, where it is slightly delayed. (This delay allows for the atria to finish contracting before the ventricles start.) Then the impulse reaches the bundle of His, passes into the bundle branches, and continues to the Purkinje fibers, where the impulse fires the ventricular myocardium.

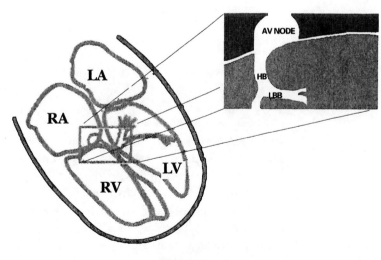

FIGURE 9.1

The presence of accessory pathways is attributed to congenitally anomalous tracts of specialized conduction tissue that bypass the A-V node or the His—Purkinje system, or both. These tracts have been named for their respective discoverers: James, Mahaim, and Kent.

As shown in Figure 9.2, James fibers bypass the A-V node by connecting the atria with the bundle of His. Mahaim fibers connect the A-V node or proximal bundle of His directly with the ventricles, producing a bypass of the His–Purkinje system. Kent fibers directly connect the atria with the ventricles, thus bypassing the A-V node *and* the His–Purkinje system.

I think I've just exhausted my multisyllabic word-use limit for this chapter. Pre-excitation syndromes are simply this: short cuts to ventricular activation. They produce EKG patterns that are not normal.

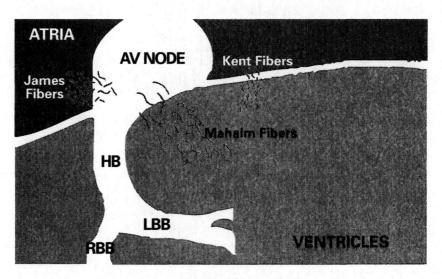

FIGURE 9.2

There are two main pre-excitation variants:

- Wolff–Parkinson–White (WPW) syndrome
- Lown–Ganong–Levine (LGL) syndrome

Both of these syndromes have upright P waves in leads I, II, and III. They each commonly have a P-R interval of less than 0.12 seconds (achieved by abnormally short accessory pathway conduction). Junctional rhythms with preceding P waves also have a P-R interval of less than 0.12 seconds. However, while junctional P waves are inverted in leads I, II, and III, pre-excitation P waves are not. The other shared factor of WPW and LGL is their potential for producing wild tachycardias.

Wolff–Parkinson–White syndrome classically has a P-R interval of less than 0.12 seconds and often a wide QRS complex (usually greater than 0.12 seconds). This wide QRS complex allows WPW to mimic bundle branch block or ventricular ectopy. However, WPW pre-excitation does not always have an abnormally short P-R interval or an abnormally wide QRS complex. About 23 percent of the time, WPW may have a P-R interval of 0.12 seconds or greater (tending to lengthen with age) and a QRS complex of less than 0.11 seconds.[1]

Diagnosis of WPW is made by looking for a *delta* wave. The delta wave is an initial slurring of the QRS complex, which represents an early and initially slow conduction through the ventricular myocardium. It is created when a supraventricular impulse travels across anomalous fibers (usually via the bundles of Kent) to bypass the A-V node, producing abnormal activation of the ventricles. In fact, as you can see in Figure 9.3, it is the delta wave that often makes the P-R interval shorter and the QRS complex wider.

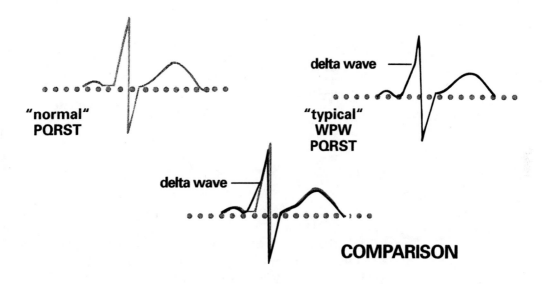

FIGURE 9.3

The size of the delta wave depends upon the percentage of ventricular activation contributed by the normal and accessory pathways, respectively. If the larger percentage is via the accessory pathway, a very short P-R interval and a wide QRS occur. If the larger percentage is contributed by the normal pathway, the QRS remains narrow (less than 0.12 seconds). The relative percentage can change frequently in the same patient, producing confusing EKGs.

Since WPW produces abnormal depolarization of the ventricles, repolarization is also abnormal. In MCL_1, deflection of the S-T segment and T wave can be opposite the QRS complex. Usually, when we see T-waves opposite from the QRS complex, we think of ischemia or ectopy. With WPW, however, this is a manifestation of the pre-excitation conduction syndrome.

There are two types of Wolff–Parkinson–White: WPW type A and WPW type B. They are differentiated by the primary direction of QRS complex deflection in MCL_1 (Figure 9.4). If the primary direction of deflection is positive (upright), it is WPW type A. If the primary direction of deflection is negative (downward), it is WPW type B.

MCL1 Lead

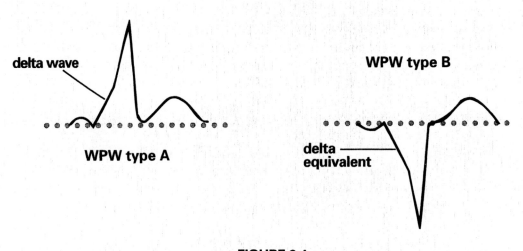

FIGURE 9.4

Technically, a delta wave is the slur on the initial, *positive* portion of the QRS complex. Therefore, true MCL_1 delta waves are only found in WPW type A. In WPW type B, the slur on the initial downward deflection of the QRS complex is negative and is called a *delta-equivalent* wave .

Since WPW type B has a primarily negative QRS deflection in MCL_1, and another manifestation of WPW is opposition of the S-T segment and T wave, WPW type B is usually accompanied by S-T elevation in MCL_1. This S-T elevation cannot be automatically attributed to ischemia. Like the S-T elevation accompanying left bundle branch block in MCL_1, WPW type B with S-T elevation in MCL_1 is not diagnostic. Either there is ischemia causing S-T elevation, or the S-T elevation is a product of the WPW.

As I mentioned earlier, WPW syndrome is usually attributed to Kent bundles (or "fibers") conducting some or all of the supraventricular impulse directly to the ventricular myocardium (Figure 9.5). Another theory about the production of WPW activation is that the James fibers and Mahaim fibers make a combined effort (Figure 9.6).

In this theory, James fibers bypass the A-V node, diverting the impulse to the proximal His bundle. There, Mahaim fibers pick up the impulse, bypassing the His–Purkinje system, and divert the impulse directly to the ventricular myocardium. In either situation the QRS complex is inscribed with an initial delta (or delta-equivalent) wave. The EKG does not show which accessory pathway route is being used.

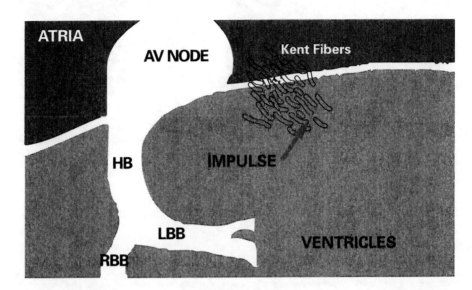

FIGURE 9.5

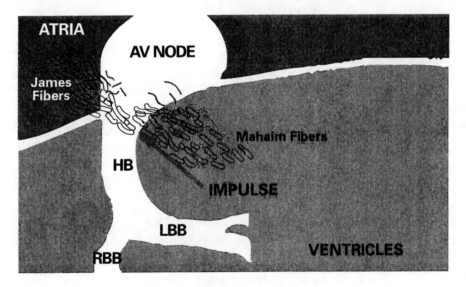

FIGURE 9.6

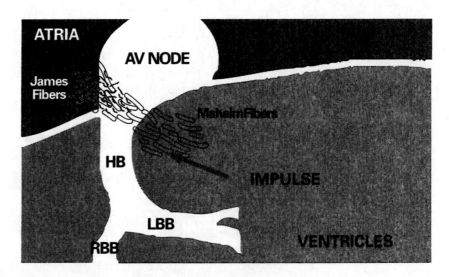

FIGURE 9.7

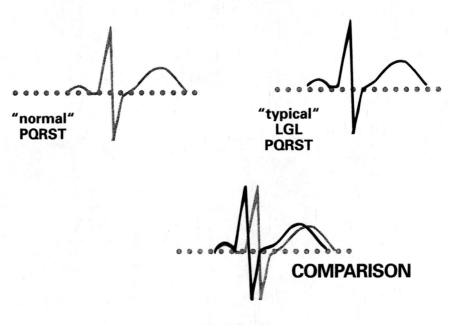

FIGURE 9.8

As shown in Figure 9.7, if the James fibers diverted *all* the supraventricular impulses to the proximal His bundle, which then conducted them normally through the His–Purkinje system, the EKG would show a very short P-R interval prior to a normally conducted QRS complex. And, unless there was an inherent bundle branch block, this would produce a QRS complex of normal duration.

This describes the pre-excitation syndrome called Lown–Ganong–Levine (LGL). LGL has not been studied as extensively as WPW. And at least one study has found that A-V node reentry was the cause of some LGL-like rhythms, not A-V nodal bypass.[2] In fact, because of the inconsistency of findings, it has been suggested that the term LGL syndrome be replaced by the term *short-PR-normal-QRS syndrome.*[1]

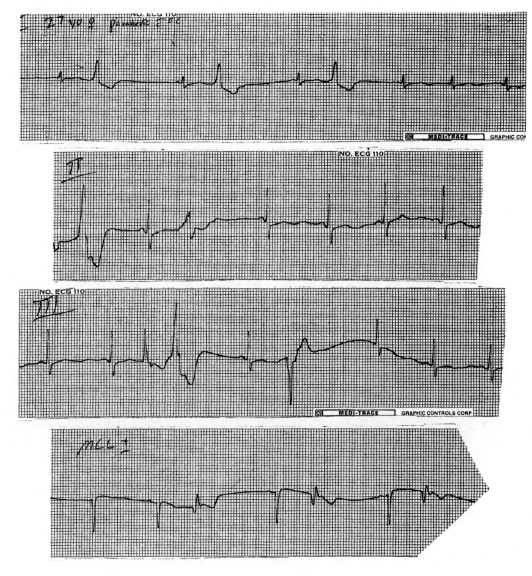

FIGURE 9.9

In any event, LGL syndrome is characterized by a short P-R interval (less than 0.12 seconds), with a QRS complex of normal duration (in the absence of a bundle branch block). The P wave that precedes or connects with the QRS complex is usually upright in leads I, II, and III. As you can see in Figure 9.8, there is no delta or delta-equivalent wave.

The EKG in Figure 9.9 is of a 27-year-old female paramedic who had consumed two strong cups of morning coffee. Her first episode of tachycardia had occurred 8 months earlier—while in a cardiology class during her paramedic training! There she experienced a sustained episode of ventricular tachycardia. In the emergency room, they discovered her pre-excitation syndrome and promptly admitted her to the hospital. During her stay, they mapped her reentry pathways, discovering 14 different ones! The only medication that would control her V tach was lidocaine. And she ended up being one of the first people in the United States to be placed on mexiletine—an oral lidocaine analog.

In Figure 9.9, her underlying rhythm is regular, with multifocal and occasionally bigeminal FLBs. The P-R interval of the underlying rhythm is 0.08 seconds and the QRS complex is less than 0.12 seconds without a delta wave. This is Lown–Ganong–Levine syndrome with FLBs.

The importance of being able to recognize pre-excitation syndromes is that these patients are prone to wild tachycardias. By "wild tachycardias," I mean tachycardias up to (and beyond) 300 beats per minute!

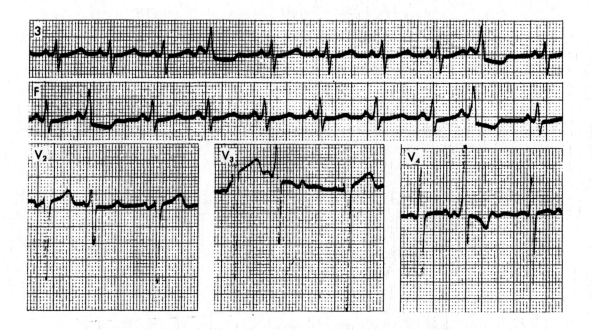

FIGURE 9.10   (Reproduced by permission of Dr. Henry J. L. Marriott, Director of Clinical Research and Education, Rogers Heart Foundation, St. Anthony's Hospital, St. Petersburg, Florida.)

Figure 9.10 shows a sinus rhythm with FLBs. Let's figure out what the FLBs are. They are each preceded by an upright, early P wave. But what happens when we compare the P-R interval of the underlying rhythm to that of each FLB? The P-R intervals of the FLBs are shorter. Whereas P-R intervals can get longer, they normally don't get shorter because A-V nodes don't suddenly conduct "better." However, if the A-V node is bypassed, the P-R interval can become shorter. If a premature atrial impulse happens to fire from an ectopic site near a congenitally anomalous pre-excitation accessory pathway and travels that pathway, the P-R interval can be shorter for the PAC that is created. Yeah, I know, "Oh, great!" If you look at leads III (3) and aVF (F) and notice that the T waves deflect opposite to the QRS complexes, you might even think the FLBs were PVCs. But when you notice the slurring of the initial part of each FLB's QRS (the delta waves), you know that these are PACs with WPW-type pre-excitation.

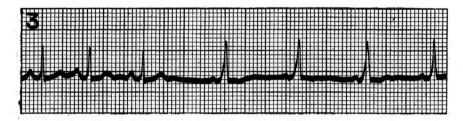

FIGURE 9.11 (Henry J. L. Marriott: *Practical Electrocardiography*, 8th ed., 1988; Williams & Wilkins, Baltimore.)

The same phenomenon can occur with an atrial escape rhythm. In Figure 9.11 you can see three sinus beats preceding a sinus pause. The atrial site that comes to the rescue is apparently near an accessory pathway. The sinus rhythm has a P-R interval of 0.13 seconds. The atrial escape has a P-R interval of 0.08 seconds and the QRS complex has developed a delta wave.

A 36-year-old male was in the ICU being treated for alcoholic hemorrhagic gastritis when his EKG began a run of wide, bizarre complexes. He remained alert and well oriented and experienced no change in his vital signs during this episode.

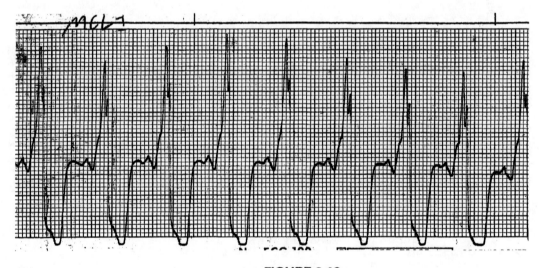

FIGURE 9.12

Figure 9.12 shows this patient's MCL$_1$ strip. It is reasonable to react to upright, wide QRS complexes with the left rabbit ear taller than the right by thinking "ventricular tachycardia!" However, closer examination reveals P waves followed by slurred delta waves at the beginning of each QRS complex. This is a classic example of type A WPW. This patient had no cardiogenic symptoms that he could recall. Since his WPW hadn't caused him clinical problems or documented episodes of tachycardia, it is probably best to refrain from treating it.

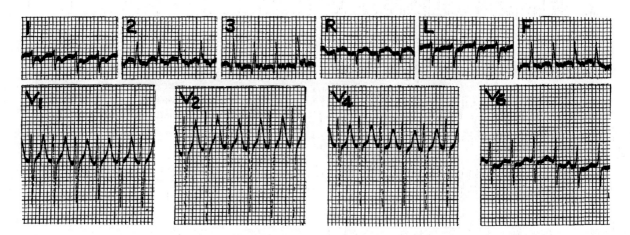

FIGURE 9.13 (Henry J. L. Marriott: *Practical Electrocardiography,*
8th ed., 1988; Williams & Wilkins, Baltimore.)

What would you call the rhythm in Figure 9.13? It looks like a
supraventricular tachycardia. The QRS complexes are well within normal
limits. The rate is too fast to see any P waves. So, the only label you can
give it is SVT.

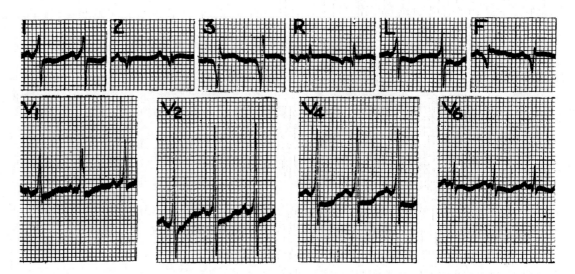

FIGURE 9.14 (Henry J. L. Marriott: *Practical Electrocardiography,*
8th ed., 1988; Williams & Wilkins, Baltimore.)

Figure 9.14 is the electrocardiogram of the same patient as Figure
9.13. It was taken after the patient (a three-week-old baby) converted to a
normal rhythm. Now what would you call it? It's not unusual to have P
waves, P-R intervals, and delta waves concealed by a supraventricular tachycardia because of the rapid rate. In fact, many paroxysmal supraventricular
tachycardias are thought to be caused by the use of accessory conduction
pathways. Once they convert to a slower rate, the morphological signs of
WPW or LGL may become visible.

Something else you need to be aware of is that the delta waves of WPW can change from beat to beat. The amount of impulse that travels the accessory path responsible for the WPW is not constant. The delta wave may become larger or smaller as the amount of impulse diverted varies. What *will* remain constant is the measurement from the beginning of the P wave to the J point. Remember that the J point is the end of the QRS complex and beginning of the T wave. You may have to hunt through other leads to clearly find the J point. But once you find it, you can compare its distance from the beginning of the P wave. And, although the delta wave/QRS complex morphology may change from beat to beat, the P-J measurement will remain constant.

Another interesting variation of WPW is that of occasional atrial impulses *without* the delta wave. A case like this might go as follows: The patient has a classic WPW sinus rhythm. Suddenly, a PVC occurs. Frequently, after a PVC, there is a sinus pause. And, just as frequently, the first impulse after the PVC is an atrial escape impulse—a site in the atria picking up the pacemaking function because the sinus pause made it think that the sinus node had failed. If this atrial escape impulse is away from the site of accessory conduction, the accessory pathway may not be used. Then the atrial impulse would travel the normal A-V node–His–Purkinje conduction route and produce a normal P-R interval and QRS complex.

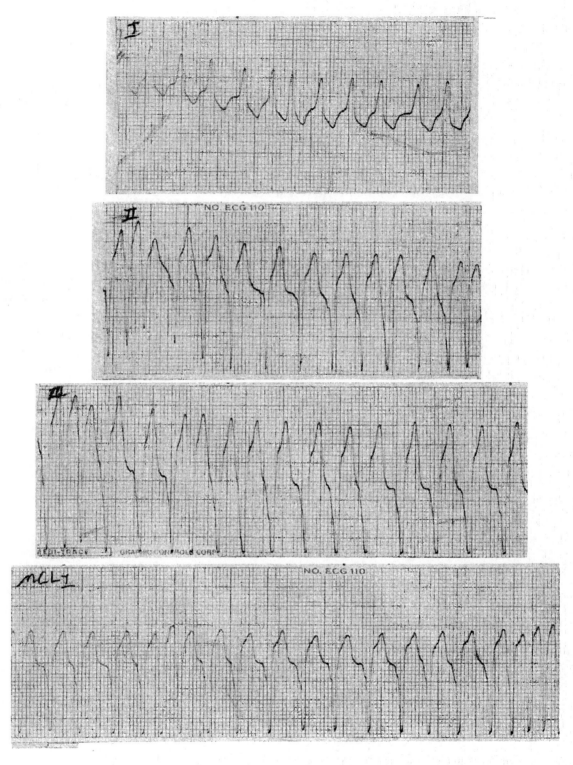

FIGURE 9.15

Some people have looked at the strip in Figure 9.15 and called it ventricular tachycardia. Remember in Chapter Eight, when we discussed rates and irregularity in tachycardias? Rates that get up to 300 beats per minute favor supraventricular tachycardia because neither the A-V node nor the ventricles generate coordinated impulses that fast. And, although all tachycardias may or may not be irregular when they are starting and stopping, a tachycardia that is persistently irregular favors a supraventricular origin of impulses—primarily atrial fibrillation, which is always irregularly irregular.

Can all atrial fibrillation get as fast as the fastest rate in Figure 9.15? Not likely. The A-V node is not normally able to conduct supraventricular impulses faster than 250 beats per minute. The A-V node was designed to *slow* impulses. In order to get a ventricular response from supraventricular impulses that goes as fast as this, there has to be one or more accessory pathways being used. Figure 9.15 shows atrial fibrillation with Wolff–Parkinson–White syndrome.

Any time you see a persistently irregular tachycardia that occasionally goes faster than 300 beats per minute, you should consider atrial fibrillation with WPW. Now, what if you see a tachycardia that is regular and has a rate right at 300 per minute? Atrial flutter with 1:1 ventricular conduction should come to mind. But, as I mentioned in the previous paragraph, it is highly unlikely that the A-V node is conducting those impulses so fast. An atrial flutter with 1:1 conduction at rates of 300 or more is probably using accessory pathways. Thus, a regular tachycardia of 300 or more beats per minute is probably atrial flutter with WPW.

Taking one last look at Figure 9.15, what type of WPW is it? MCL_1 shows a negative QRS complex deflection, making it WPW type B.

Our next case is that of a 49-year-old woman named Frieda, who boarded a flight at LaGuardia airport in New York City. During the flight to Los Angeles, she got up and grabbed hold of a flight attendant who also happened to be a registered nurse. She said, "I think I'm gonna pass out." A nearby passenger, a big guy who happened to be a respiratory therapist, overheard Frieda's complaint. He helped the flight attendant walk Frieda to the back of the plane to lie down. Soon after they got her supine and made her comfortable, Frieda had a syncopal episode. They happened to notice that her pupils had dilated, and then they realized she had become apneic and pulseless.

The respiratory therapist did the initial four stair-stepping breaths of mouth-to-mouth resuscitation, just as he had been trained to. Suddenly Frieda woke up. She looked about and asked, "What's going on?" Then she immediately lost consciousness again.

Once again, the flight attendant RN and the respiratory therapist noticed that Frieda's pupils had become dilated, she wasn't breathing, and she didn't have a pulse. Once again the respiratory therapist did the initial four stair-stepping breaths of mouth-to-mouth resuscitation, and Frieda woke up.

She soon proceeded to have a third syncopal episode while supine. This time, however, they thought they could feel a very rapid, very weak carotid pulse. But since she was apneic again, the big guy gave her the four breaths and woke her up again.

When the flight attendant was finally able to break away and inform the pilot of what was going on, he made an unscheduled landing at Denver's Stapleton International Airport. The paramedic stationed at the airport responded in the emergency medical golf cart, meeting the aircraft as it pulled up to the gate. All eyes were on the paramedic as he carried his equipment to the back of the aircraft. Upon hearing the story related by the registered nurse and respiratory therapist, the paramedic turned to Frieda and said, "Well, let's get you off the plane and figure out what's going on." To which Frieda replied, "Oh, no. I have a job interview in Los Angeles. I can't get off here!"

Not to be daunted, the paramedic was about to begin his gently nudging negotiating strategy for sick patients refusing care, when the pilot stepped between him and Frieda. The pilot engaged Frieda in a hammerlock wrestling hold, lifted her up, and marched her off the plane (all the while mumbling something about it costing ten thousand dollars-per-minute to make unscheduled landings at international airports)! Quickly grabbing his gear, the paramedic scurried after the patient and pilot. Once patient and paramedic were gently tossed off the aircraft, the pilot dove back into the cockpit and the door swooshed closed behind them in preparation for take-off.

As soon as she was settled in the terminal, Frieda threw the adult equivalent of a temper tantrum. With loud, rapid speech and much gesticulation, Frieda demanded that someone from the airline call her boyfriend in Los Angeles to let him know what was going on. As a representative went to accomplish her demands, the paramedic convinced Frieda to let him evaluate her medical condition.

As soon as the paramedic had finished obtaining the EKG in Figure 9.16, the airline representative returned and said, "Excuse me, Miss Frieda's boyfriend is on the phone and has vital medical information he says you should know about before taking care of her."

Over the phone, Frieda's boyfriend explained that Frieda had a hysterical personality disorder "and there's nothing medically wrong with her! Please just give her a Valium and put her back on the plane—she's got a job interview to get to!"

Well, the paramedic looked at Frieda's short P-R interval. He looked at the delta wave barely visible in lead III. He considered the EKG findings in combination with the history provided by the respiratory therapist and the RN flight attendant. And he realized that Valium was unlikely to be the therapeutic drug of choice for Frieda and her episodes of WPW tachycardia. Finally, since the Valium-prescribing boyfriend wasn't physically present, the paramedic decided to terminate the phone call, initiate oxygen, start an IV line, and send Frieda to the hospital by ambulance.

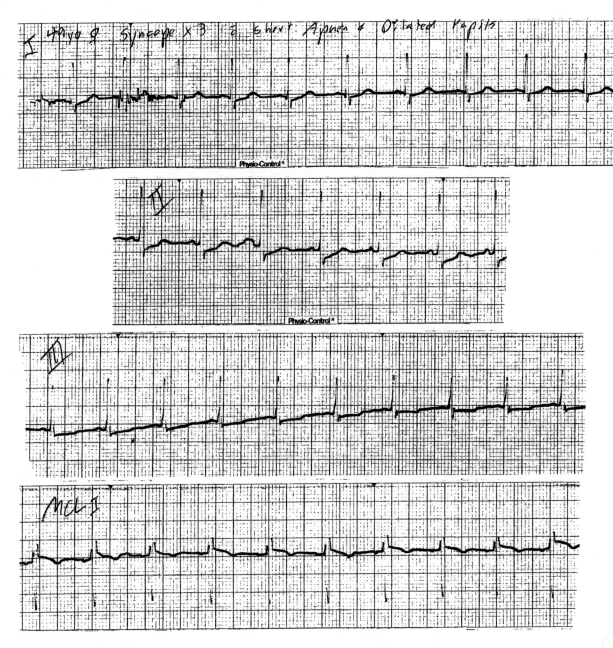

FIGURE 9.16

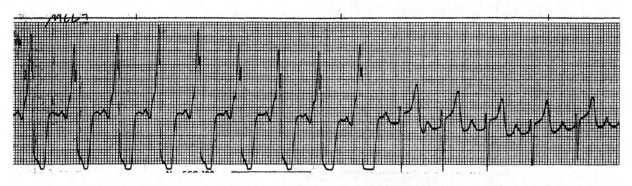

FIGURE 9.17

Remember the EKG from the alcoholic being treated in the ICU? (Figure 9.12.) Figure 9.17 shows his pathways changing back to normal. When our workshop audiences see this strip they are often confused. The beginning looks so radically different than the end. Physiologically, the only difference is that the beginning uses the anomalous pathway and the end conducts via the normal pathway. There is virtually no difference in rate—consequently, no change in the patient's signs or symptoms. Sometimes, when assessing a complex EKG, it is helpful to focus on segments and then relate them to the whole strip.

SUMMARY

Pre-excitation syndromes such as WPW and LGL are caused by congenitally anomalous pathways of conduction fibers within the heart. These patients usually have normal cardiac rhythms. Their hearts don't necessarily use these pathways all the time. The only time they get into trouble is when one of their pathways sets up a re-entry cycle that results in tachycardia.

REFERENCES

1. Sherf, L., and Neufeld, N. H.: *The Pre-excitation Syndrome: Facts and Theories.* Yorke Medical Books, New York, 1978.
2. Benditt, D. G., et al., Characteristics of atrioventricular conduction and the spectrum of arrhythmias in Lown–Ganong–Levine syndrome. *Circulation* 1978:57,454.

CHAPTER 10

Pacemaker Rhythms

There are almost as many different pacemakers on today's market as there are software programs available for personal computers. These pacemakers have all kinds of "lights, bells, whistles" and multiple high-tech features. They often are small enough to fit into a control box the size of a postage stamp and aren't very much thicker. The days of being able to look at a patient's chest and find the can-of-chewing-tobacco-like battery sewn beneath the skin below the right clavicle are history. And determining pacemaker placement based on that finding is too. Consequently, it is well beyond the scope of this book to discuss in detail the intricacies and complexities of the various types of electrical devices that may be found implanted in your patients.

In general, pacemakers and automatic implanted cardioverter-defibrillators (AICDs) are implanted in patients with impaired electrical activation of their heart muscle. A pacemaker is designed to replace or supplement the patient's natural cardiac impulse generation. AICDs are designed to sense the onset of ventricular tachycardia or ventricular fibrillation and immediately deliver an electrical shock to interrupt these life-threatening arrhythmias.

A properly functioning pacemaker has two primary tasks. First, it must know that there is a need to produce an electrical cardiac stimulus when one is naturally lacking. That is, it must *sense* the need to fire a stimulus. Second, when a pacemaker fires, it must stimulate the heart muscle to depolarize and contract. This is referred to as *capture*. So a properly functioning pacemaker must sense and capture.

We used to be able to easily assess whether pacemakers were functioning appropriately with a routine electrocardiogram. These days, assessment of pacemaker function is greatly dependent upon the ability to decipher codes that are found on the pacemaker patient's wallet identification card or medic alert bracelet. Few prehospital care providers have this code-deciphering training. Because of this, when treating a pacemaker patient, I strongly recommend that you focus your attention more on clinical assessment than on electrocardiographic assessment. Of course, there are some very specific exceptions to this recommendation. These exceptions are the pacemaker function assessments that can be made in the field. I call these exceptions *Pacemaker Principles.*

Pacemaker principle 1: If your patient has a pacemaker, is bradycardic or hypoperfusing, and you don't see any pacemaker spikes on the electrocardiogram, the patient's pacemaker is probably not working. Treat the patient according to standard ACLS bradycardia protocols. If you have an external pacemaker, engage it!

Pacemaker principle 2: If your pacemaker patient is in a wide complex tachycardia, it makes no difference what the pacemaker is doing or not doing. You need to treat the wide complex tachycardia.

Pacemaker principle 3: If the pacemaker patient's heart rate is somewhere within normal range but the patient's perfusion is inadequate, electrocardiographic complications are probably not to blame for the hypoperfusion. You need to assess for other causes of hypoperfusion and treat the patient for those. Leave the patient's heart rate alone.

Pacemaker principle 4: If the patient has a pacemaker, has a reasonable heart rate, and is perfusing adequately, don't worry about the pacemaker!

When assessing the EKG of patients with pacemakers, as with any other electrocardiographic information, one lead is not enough. Pacemaker spikes are not always visible in all leads. Figure 10.1 shows the V leads of a paced rhythm. As you can see, the spikes are only clearly distinguishable in leads V_3, V_4, and V_5. If someone were truly astute (and ran MCL_6), they may note the spike initiating the QRS complex in V_6. But if all you looked at was MCL_1, you wouldn't recognize this as a paced rhythm.

In Figure 10.2 you see a strip of MCL_1 with upright QRS complexes. At the beginning of each QRS is the faintly inscribed left epicardial pacemaker spike. Of the many potential causes of an upright QRS complex in MCL_1 (right bundle branch block, posterior wall AMI, WPW type A, right ventricular enlargement, and others), one is a left epicardial pacemaker.

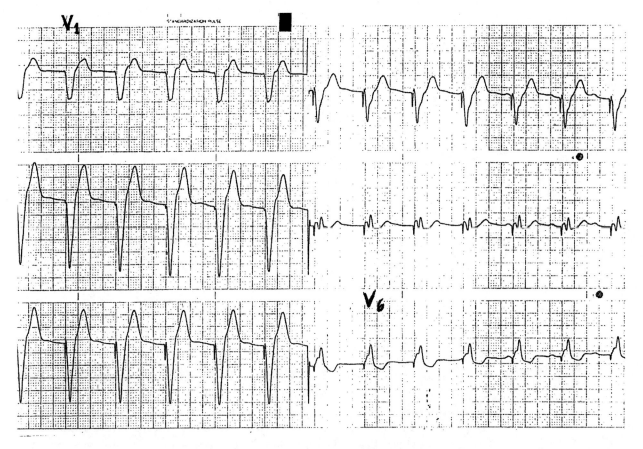

FIGURE 10.1

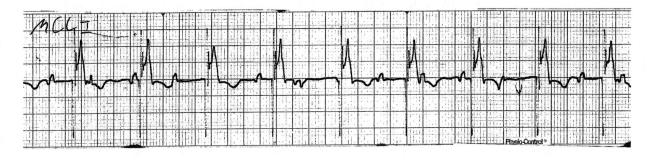

FIGURE 10.2

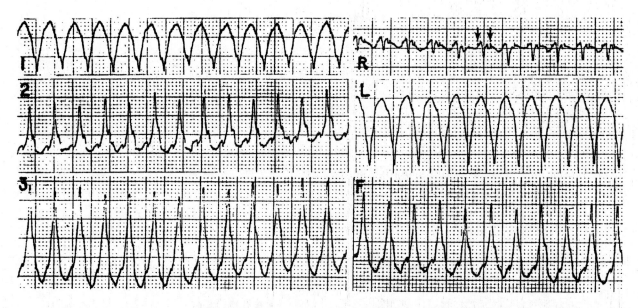

FIGURE 10.3 (Henry J. L. Marriott: *Practical Electrocardiography*, 8th ed., 1988; Williams & Wilkins, Baltimore.)

Figure 10.3 is the EKG of a patient who walked into the emergency room complaining of a "fluttering" in his chest. The patient was alert, had a blood pressure of 100/60, and had this wide complex tachycardia. When they saw his EKG, the emergency department team considered his blood pressure (over 100 systolic) and decided that this must be supraventricular tachycardia with aberrant ventricular conduction.

Does this case sound at all familiar? It should. This is the runaway pacemaker case presented in Chapter Eight—the fatal runaway pacemaker case. This gentleman's pacemaker is firing at a rate of 440 a minute, and the spikes are only visible in aVR. There are two spikes to each QRS complex. This is because the patient's myocardium is only able to respond to every other spike, half the pacemaker rate or 220 beats per minute. If the pacemaker spikes had been discovered earlier (*before* the Verapamil, lidocaine, Bretylium, and over 30 consecutive unsuccessful cardioversions at 360 watt-seconds), he may have survived. The tre0atment of a runaway pacemaker is, as Dr. Marriott puts it, to isolate "the offending pulse generator."

The EKG in Figure 10.4 is that of a 78-year-old male who had an atraumatic syncopal episode, resulting in a call to 911. Upon our arrival, Ralph was alert, well oriented, and denied all complaints (of course, he didn't remember "fainting"). His blood pressure was 110 by palpation. He had a pulse of 84 and a respiratory rate of 16. His skin was warm, dry, and pink. His only complaint was that, for some unknown reason, we were there to take him to the hospital and he didn't feel the need to go. Ralph's electrocardiogram shows an A-V sequential pacemaker. This means he has electrodes pacing *both* his atria and his ventricles.

In most people, the extra circulation produced by contraction of the atria is not necessary to maintain reasonable perfusion. People with chronic atrial fibrillation don't have coordinated atrial contractions. Yet they perfuse just fine (until some *other* problem occurs). However, if someone has A-V valve problems, such as mitral stenosis, a coordinated atrial "kick" (contraction) becomes infinitely more important to their overall cardiac output. Without a healthy valve to prevent valvular regurgitation (retrograde flow of blood during ventricular contraction), ventricular ejection becomes severely impaired. With the addition of forceful atrial contraction, ventricular filling is improved, thus improving ventricular ejection, despite the continued presence of valvular regurgitation.

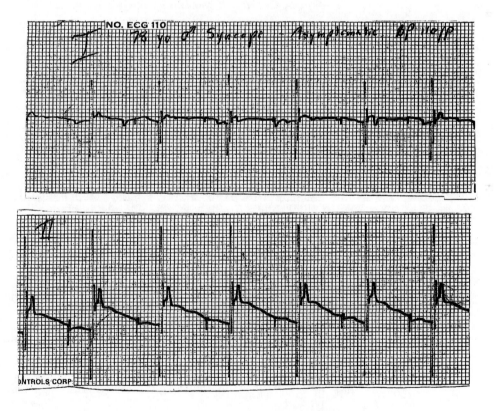

FIGURE 10.4 *continued on page 172*
continued on page 172

Consequently, these people need two pacemakers: an atrial pacemaker electrode to produce regular, coordinated atrial contractions, and a ventricular electrode to produce regular, coordinated ventricular contractions. Thus, they need an *A-V sequential pacemaker.*

It would appear that Ralph's A-V sequential pacemaker is capturing effectively because there are P waves after the atrial pacer spikes and QRS complexes after the ventricular pacer spikes. We are unable to tell from this electrocardiogram if the pacemaker is sensing. The only way we would know that Ralph's pacemaker was sensing would be if his natural, intrinsic pacemaker took over and fired a couple of beats. If the pacemaker spikes stopped during that period of naturally generated beats, we would know that the pacemaker was sensing the need *not* to fire. When the natural pacemaker failed and the pacemaker spikes resumed, we would know that the pacemaker was sensing properly.

Is it a problem that we can't tell if Ralph's pacemaker is sensing? No. Pacemaker principle 4: If the patient has a pacemaker, has a reasonable heart rate, and is perfusing adequately, don't worry about the pacemaker! Certainly, we had to convince Ralph to let us take him in for a "checkup" to try to determine the cause of his syncope. But we found him with adequate mentation, sufficient blood pressure, and a reasonable heart rate. Thus, our treatment was based upon his clinical assessment, not that of his electrocardiogram. He received oxygen by nasal cannula, a volume-expanding IV fluid run at TKO, and a gentle ride to the hospital.

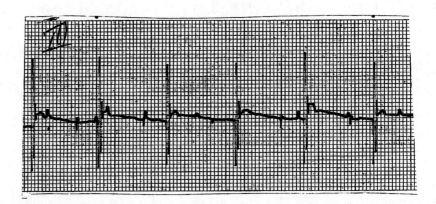

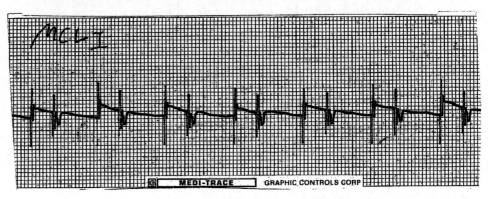

FIGURE 10.4 *continued*

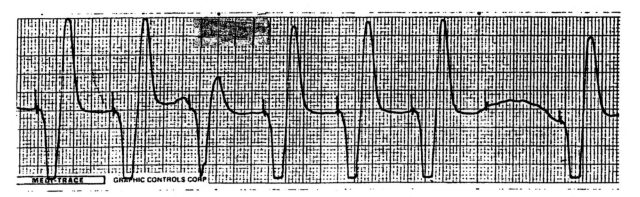

FIGURE 10.5

Figure 10.5 is that of an interesting patient. The full story that accompanies this patient's EKG will be presented in Chapter Twelve. For now, let me just point out that this is a paced rhythm where capture is occasionally ineffective.

What is the cause of the change in morphology for the third QRS complex? It's a fusion beat. The patient's natural pacemaker fired an impulse that reached the ventricles at the same time as that of the pacemaker.

Fusion beats occur when two (or more) impulses activate the same part of the heart at the same time. This combined activation produces a complex that is grossly dissimilar to the others in the strip, yet often contains similar recognizable features. Fusion can occur in the atria, in the ventricles, and with all types of ectopy (especially end-diastolic PVCs such as those seen in Figure 8.20). Fusion may occur during V tach, accelerated idioventricular rhythms, any escape rhythms, and paced rhythms.

Not only are fusion beats *not* unusual in paced patients, Dr. Marriott calls the pacemaker "a splendid fusion factory." PVCs may also occur during a paced rhythm. Both PVCs and fusion are considered normal occurrences and are not necessarily causes for concern.

I include Figure 10.5 here to illustrate pacemaker principle 3: If the pacemaker patient's heart rate is somewhere within the normal range, but the patient manifests signs and symptoms of inadequate perfusion, electrocardiographic complications are probably not to blame. You need to assess for other causes of hypoperfusion and treat the patient for those. There is nothing wrong with this patient's pacemaker. Granted, capture is occasionally ineffective, but the pacemaker spikes are regular and occur at an appropriate rate. Some other dysfunction is producing this patient's inadequate perfusion.

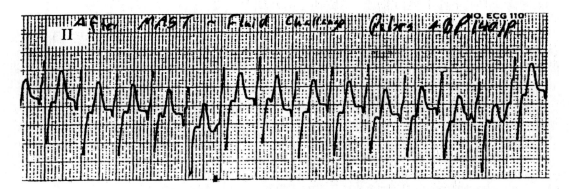

FIGURE 10.6

The patient in Figure 10.6 happened to be apneic and pulseless during the strip you see. CPR and ACLS were performed. After administration of a fluid challenge and the inflation of MAST trousers, this patient converted to a sinus tachycardia, with a blood pressure of 140 by palpation. Figure 10.6 is the EKG strip obtained during this tachycardia.

As you can see, there are no pacemaker spikes present. The pacemaker is appropriately sensing the natural pacemaker's generation of a tachycardia and not firing.

SUMMARY

Because pacemaker technology has become tremendously refined and extensive, a prehospital provider would be hard-pressed to keep up. It is probably better to take the pacemaker principles to heart and act accordingly than to try to stay abreast of pacemaker development. Another good strategy in keeping with the information presented in this chapter: know how and when to use your external (transcutaneous) pacemaker equipment, if your patients are lucky enough for you to have one.

CHAPTER 11

Infarct Area Identification Patterns

In the emergency room, many patients who are admitted with the diagnosis of "rule out myocardial infarction" turn out *not* to have one. This is because there are numerous situations that produce chest pain or chest discomfort that have nothing to do with infarction of the myocardium. But since definitive signs of myocardial infarction (MI) are often hidden or delayed, the potential of infarction must always be addressed.

Generally speaking, the suspicion of cardiac ischemia and myocardial infarction should be based primarily upon history, not upon physical examination or EKG findings. A normal electrocardiogram does *not* rule out myocardial infarction. EKG changes may be late to develop. Sometimes they take *days* to appear on the electrocardiogram. Any time the clinical impression suggests potential acute myocardial infarction, treat the patient as if acute myocardial infarction has occurred.

The ability to obtain a thorough medical history is a vastly underrated skill. History taking is often poorly performed by prehospital and inhospital providers alike. If medical practitioners were to truly listen to patients, they would discover that patients tell us precisely what is wrong with them most of the time! But most of us don't *listen* to our patients. We take information from patients and immediately put it through preset history "filters" to try and "sift out" a diagnosis. Often we miss crucial clues because the information we've already sifted has us pointed toward a different diagnosis.

In addition to developing better listening skills, we also need to examine the questions we frequently ask patients in our attempts to elicit more information. Chapter Five contained some examples of how often we lead, limit, and confuse patients with the wording of our questions. The techniques mentioned there can never be reviewed too often.

Initiation of thrombolytic therapy, however, depends on EKG confirmation of myocardial infarction. When a coronary artery becomes occluded, the affected area of myocardium beyond the occlusion produces electrocardiographic changes. These changes can be seen in the leads that have positive electrodes located over the part of the heart that is infarcting. Thus, when EKG signs of ischemia, injury, or infarction appear in certain leads, it becomes possible to reasonably predict what areas of the heart are becoming damaged and thus what vessels in the heart may be occluded.

Let's quickly review the myocardial structures normally supplied by each coronary artery.[1]

The right coronary artery (RCA) normally supplies:

- SA node (50 to 60 percent of the time)
- Right atrium
- Right ventricular wall

Eighty-five to 90 percent of the time, the posterior descending right coronary artery (RCA) also supplies:

- A-V node
- Proximal His bundle
- One-half to two-thirds of the posterior ventricular septum
- Left ventricle's posteromedial papillary muscle
- Half of the diaphragmatic surface of the heart
- A portion of the posterior fascicle of the left bundle branch

The left anterior descending coronary artery (LAD) supplies:

- Most of the ventricular septum
- Anterior, lateral, and apical left ventricular walls
- Anterolateral left papillary muscle
- Most of the right and left bundle branches
- Anterior fascicle of the left bundle branch

The left circumflex coronary artery (CCA) supplies:

- SA node (40 to 45 percent of the time)
- Left atrium
- Lateral and posterior ventricular walls
- A portion of the posterior fascicle of the left bundle branch

As mentioned in Chapter Four, you can see why it is so much more dangerous to have a posterior hemiblock—a blocked posterior fascicle. Two major arteries supply this fascicle with nutrients and oxygenated blood. In order to block this fascicle, you have to have occlusion or damage to both the right and circumflex coronary arteries. Occlusion of only one artery (the left anterior descending) is all that is required to injure the anterior fascicle.

There is a triad of EKG signs (Marriott calls them "indicative changes") that indicate myocardial ischemia, injury, or infarction. The presence of inverted T waves indicates ischemia and is considered to be a *reversible* sign. S-T segment elevation is produced by injury to the myocardium and is also considered reversible. The development of new Q waves, however, indicates irreversible death of myocardial tissue—myocardial infarction.

The first sign of ischemia is T wave inversion, also known as "flipped" T waves. This is when the T wave is opposite to what would be considered normal for each specific lead. As you can see on page 178, not all leads normally have upright T waves. In MCL_1, the T wave is normally negative. So an upright T wave in MCL_1 is considered to be flipped and could be indicative of ischemic alterations in the electrocardiogram.

As ischemia progresses to injury, S-T segments in the facing leads (those located over the infarcted area) begin to elevate from the baseline. The leads opposite to the infarcted area may contain what are called *reciprocal* EKG changes (in this case, depressed S-T segments). Some experts consider reciprocal changes to be indicative of even greater injury, rather than simply a reciprocation of changes in the facing leads.

If the injury progresses to myocardial tissue death, wide (and sometimes deep) Q waves may occur. Any Q wave that measures 0.03 seconds wide or wider is considered to be wide enough to indicate an infarction.

It is important to remember that all three of these signs should only serve to increase a suspicion of MI *already established* by the patient's history. Absence of Q waves does not rule out MI. Q waves may develop quickly or may not be seen for several days. Likewise, the presence of Q waves does not rule *in* MI. There are a multitude of noninfarction conditions that may produce Q waves. These include anterior and posterior hemiblocks, right or left ventricular hypertrophy, pulmonary embolism, pneumonia, even acute pancreatitis.[2]

The actual names used for the location of infarctions seem to vary from author to author, so it isn't reasonable to be dogmatic about it. Hearts don't have clearly defined boundaries between anterior, posterior, lateral, and inferior areas. Any single infarction may easily involve more than one area. Simultaneously occurring, *separate* infarctions can alter each other's patterns so that neither pattern can be clearly observed. Keeping these warnings clearly in mind, let us now discuss the most common patterns observed in anterior, lateral, inferior, and posterior infarctions.

> *Anterior infarction* is identified by indicative changes (Q waves, S-T elevation, or T wave inversion) in leads I, aVL, and the mid-precordial leads (V_2, V_3, V_4, and V_5).

> *Lateral infarctions* are identified by indicative changes in leads I, aVL, V_5, and V_6.

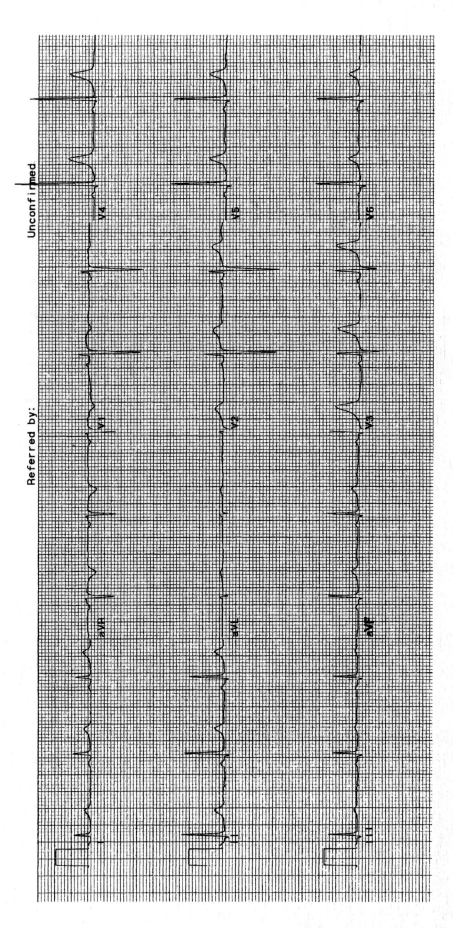

FIGURE 11.1 Normal Direction of T Waves: Positive deflection in leads I, II, III, V_3 to V_6. Negative deflection in leads aVR, V_1, and V_2. May normally vary in leads III, aVF, V_1, and V_2.

Inferior infarctions are identified by indicative changes in leads II, III, and aVF.

Posterior infarctions are identified differently from the rest. We use leads on the opposite side of the heart from the infarction, and look for reciprocal changes—tall and/or broad R waves in V_1 and V_2.

Patterns for Recognizing Infarctions

Indicative changes (Q waves, S-T elevation, T wave inversion)

    Anterior MI: leads I, aVL, (V_2, V_3, V_4, V_5

    Lateral MI: leads I, aVL, V_5, V_6

    Inferior MI: leads II, III, aVF

Reciprocal changes (tall and/or broad R waves)

    Posterior MI: leads V_1 and V_2

To assist you in the field, I've included a chart of patterns for anterior, lateral, and inferior infarctions here and in the appendix of this text. Photocopy the chart and reduce it to fit into your pocket reference book, or affix it to your monitor to have it handy.

Figures 11.2, 11.3, 11.4, and 11.5 are examples of common myocardial infarction patterns.

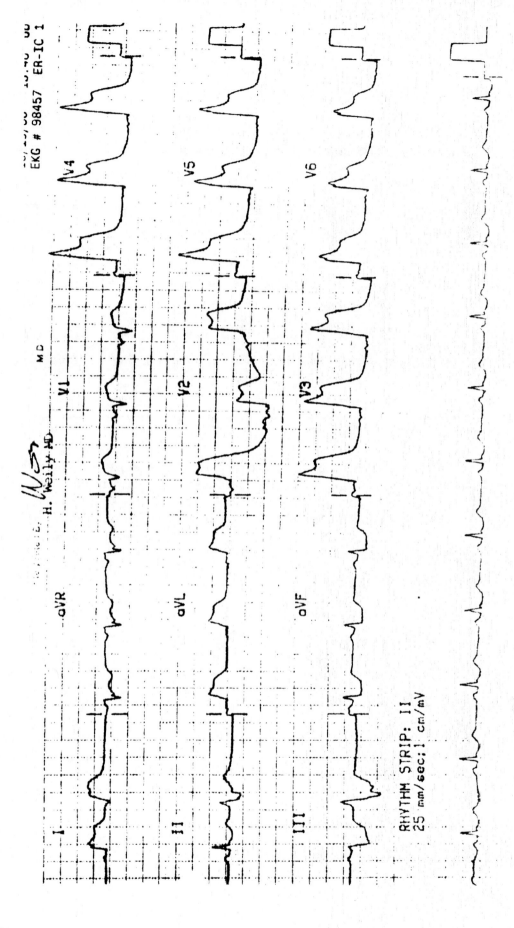

FIGURE 11.2 Normal sinus rhythm. Signs of a large anterior wall myocardial infarction (S-T segment elevation in I, aVL, V$_{1-6}$). S-T segments like these are often called "tombstone" S-T segments—and for a good reason.

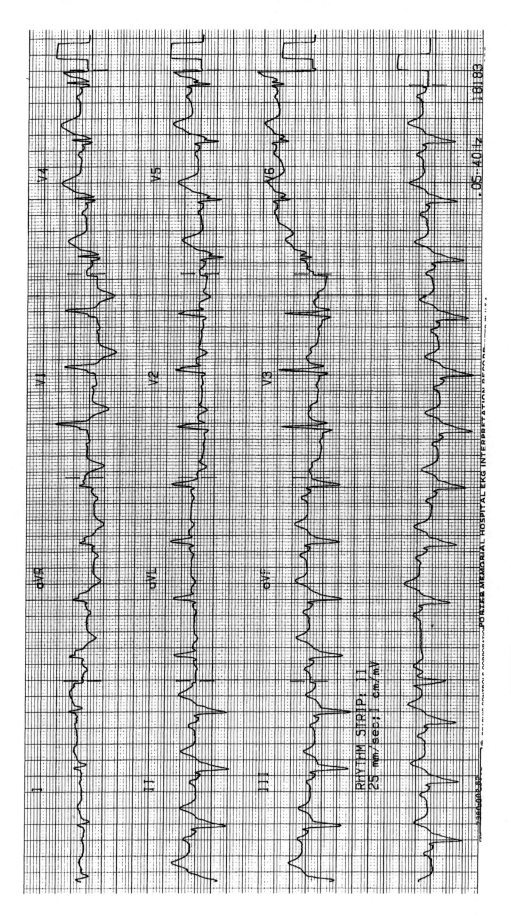

FIGURE 11.3 Normal sinus rhythm with right bundle branch block, pathologic left axis deviation, left anterior hemiblock, and signs of anterior wall myocardial infarction (S-T elevation in I, aVR, and V_{2-6}).

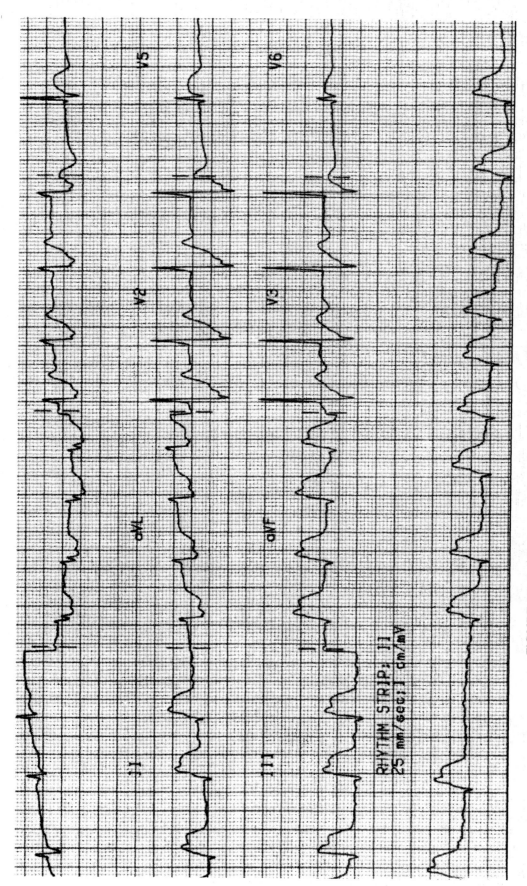

FIGURE 11.4 Atrial fibrillation with a slow ventricular response and indicative signs of an inferior wall myocardial infarction (S-T segment elevation and q waves in II, III, aVF). There are also indicative signs of a lateral wall myocardial infarction (S-T segment elevation in V_4, V_5, V_6) and S-T segment depression in V_1, V_2, and V_3. The bottom line is that this patient has a very sick heart.

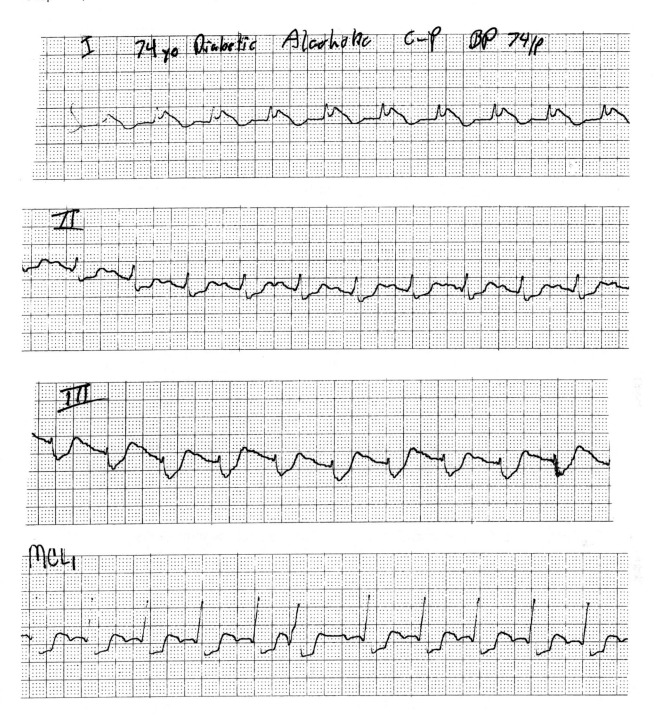

FIGURE 11.5 Normal sinus rhythm with prolonged P-R interval (0.22 seconds), occasional PACs, and signs of a posterior-lateral wall myocardial infarction (tall, broad R wave in MCL₁ and S-T segment elevation in I). He also has S-T segment depression in II and III. When combined with the blood pressure of 74 by palpation, this patient also has a very sick heart.

There are also some subtler signs of myocardial infarction or ischemia. These are often transient and occur very early in the course of an infarction. If they are going to be observed on the patient's electrocardiogram at all, the prehospital care provider will most often be the one with the best chance to identify and document them. These subtle signs consist of a *hyperacute* R wave and a *horizontality* of the S-T segment.

A hyperacute R wave is one that becomes taller for a brief period of time, and then returns to normal.

The normal S-T segment leaves the QRS complex at the junction point (the J point) and gently blends into the T wave. If, instead, the S-T segment is radically flat (horizontal) and at a sharp angle to the T wave, this is one of the earliest signs of ischemia or infarction.

Again, both of these signs are transient, usually lasting only a few minutes. Thus, if you see one or both of these signs, it is helpful to report them to the receiving physician.

Occasionally, infarctions can be identified with specific arrhythmias. Anterior myocardial infarctions tend to cause conduction problems in the structures supplied by the anterior descending coronary artery. Anterior hemiblock, bundle branch blocks, and type II A-V blocks are not uncommon. Inferior myocardial infarctions are often associated with bradycardias and type I A-V blocks.

SUMMARY

Various current research projects seem to indicate that paramedics can dramatically shorten the time between onset of an infarction and the administration of "clot busters." Paramedics have been able to accurately identify patients with myocardial infarction and initiate the checklist used to include or exclude them as candidates for thrombolytic intervention. Some are administering thrombolytic therapy in the field.

As this text is being written, the question yet to be answered is, whether it makes a difference. Does the savings of 45 minutes, or even an hour, actually affect the patient's long-term recovery and life-style prognoses? Watch the research literature for the answer to this question.

REFERENCES

1. Hurst, J. W., ed., *The Heart, Arteries and Veins*, 7th ed., 1990; McGraw-Hill Book Co., New York.

2. Marriott, Henry J. L.: *Practical Electrocardiography*, 8th ed., 1988; Williams & Wilkins, Baltimore.

CHAPTER 12

Wild and Crazy EKGs

In this chapter we're going to explore a collection of "wild and crazy EKGs" (just like the chapter title suggests). These cases are not presented just for fun! Although they *are* a lot of fun, these are unusual cases that present us with wonderful opportunities to learn. Some of them are cases I experienced firsthand. Others are cases that were shared with me by a variety of professional care providers I've met throughout my years in EMS. If you recognize a case that you shared with me (and you haven't been previously acknowledged in this text), please insert your name in the following blank space: Mike, Syd, and Charly heartily thank_____for benefiting others by contributing this valuable case study to the cardiology workshops and this text! Seriously, though, this text (and the workshops that gave birth to it) would not have been possible without the generosity and talent of a number of paramedics, nurses, and physicians. Thank you all.

Lets get to it, shall we?

We were dispatched to a "syncopal episode." When we arrived at the patient's apartment, the first thing we noticed was that the place was *trashed*! Stuff was everywhere; knocked over, ripped up, and falling off the walls. Our patient was a 54-year-old gentleman named Mr. McDougal. We found Mr. McDougal kneeling on his kitchen floor with bits of dirt and parts of a potted plant hanging from his Santa Claus-type, salt-and-pepper beard. He looked miserable. He was hyperventilating a bit and had tears rolling down his face.

"Gawd, what happened?" I asked him.

"This is the worst day of my entire life!" he exclaimed. Mr. McDougal then proceeded to tell us about his day.

He had taken a bus downtown to get a bite to eat. On his way from the bus to his favorite diner, he was mugged by a couple of boys. They knocked him to the ground and stole his wallet and watch. But what he found most upsetting was that they also took his pocket change, which meant he had to beg money from strangers to get the next bus back home. When he managed to get home, he found his apartment ransacked. While he was being mugged, he had been burglarized!

Mr. McDougal told us he had been married for 22 years. He and his wife, Marion, were the kind of couple that always did everything together. They never had separate vacations, never were apart. Well, Marion's father had died just the week before and she was in Chicago for the funeral. This was the first time in their 22-year marriage that Mr. McDougal and his wife had been apart. When he got home from being mugged and found their little apartment burglarized, he called Marion on the telephone. As he was telling her about the whole, horrible ordeal, his wife burst into tears on the other end of the line and the phone went dead.

That was the final straw—it was just too much. He described acute anxiousness and rapid breathing before feeling "faint" and falling into a small table (the one that once supported the plant now hanging from his beard). Mr. McDougal's description of what happened sounded like a frantic hyperventilation episode productive of syncope. As you can imagine, I was pretty upset for him and easily understood how his situation could have produced emotional syncope. I helped him pluck the plant from his beard and performed my exam as he pulled himself together.

His pulse was 80 and regular, his blood pressure 140/100. He originally looked a little pale and had a deep respiratory rate of about 36. After talking to him for a bit, though, his respiratory rate calmed down to 18, his skin color pinked up, and he began to look much better. He had no physical complaints. He hadn't been physically injured during the mugging and hadn't had chest pain or nausea before or after the syncopal episode. And his chief complaint became, "What do I do now?"

Normally, after I've successfully treated a patient's emotional hyperventilation with counseling and reassurance, I'm not inclined to take them to a hospital. But Mr. McDougal had been psychologically devastated. He had been robbed, burglarized, his home was a mess, he was all alone for the first time in his life, and I didn't want to just leave him there. So I said, "Why don't we give you a ride to the hospital? You can get some help finding a place to stay for the night, and maybe social services can arrange assistance for cleaning your apartment." Mr. McDougal agreed that help would be welcomed and walked out to the ambulance with us.

Once on our way to the hospital, I figured that I might as well run an EKG on him. Mr. McDougal's episode had clearly been one of emotional hyperventilation, he had no other signs or symptoms of a cardiac episode, and the event appeared completely resolved. But, after all, he was 54 years old, so what would it hurt to run an EKG? Figure 12.1 was his EKG while en route to the hospital.

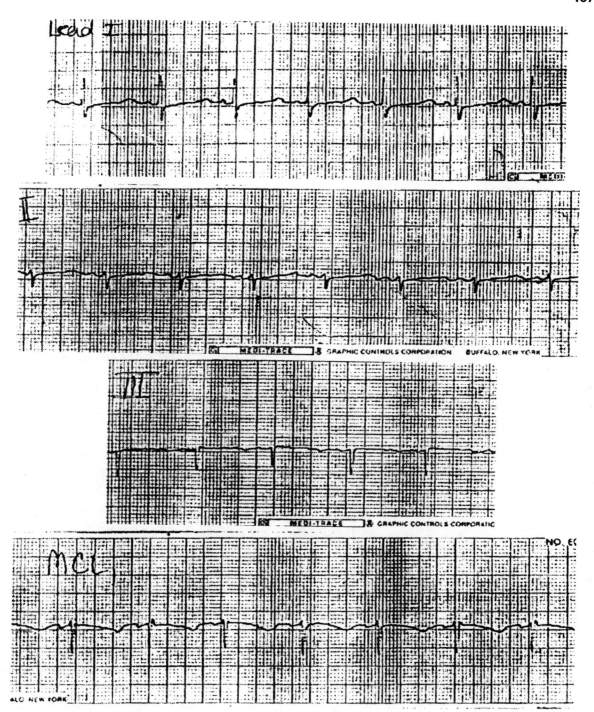

FIGURE 12.1

As you can see, Mr. McDougal had a regular, sinus rhythm with a pathologic left axis deviation. So he had a left anterior hemiblock. His QRS complexes were well within normal limits and he had no ectopy. But, while observing for S-T segment abnormalities, I noticed that he appeared to have rather long Q-T segments.

After watching me run his EKG, Mr. McDougal asked, "Well, how's the heart?" I told him it looked pretty good, but that he might have some electrolytes "out of whack." Then he asked, "Could that come from drinking a lot of water?"

"Why do you ask me that?"

"'cause I drink a lot of water."

"Well, how much is 'a lot of water'?"

"Oh. I don't know. About 12, maybe 14 quarts a day. I take Mellaril and it makes my mouth real dry."

At about that point, I decided it might be a neat thing to draw some blood samples and put an IV in Mr. McDougal. I still wasn't convinced that he had had more than an emotional hyperventilation and syncope. But, being concerned about those long Q-T intervals, I wanted to make sure he would get a good medical checkup before his social service referral.

We were transporting Mr. McDougal without lights and sirens, and where I worked at that time we didn't call in reports for nonemergent patients. During the rest of our trip in, I discovered no other abnormal findings or surprising bits of information. As we backed up to the emergency room door, I was about to discontinue the monitor when Mr. McDougal suddenly became unresponsive and had a little seizure. Figure 12.2 is what his EKG looked like then.

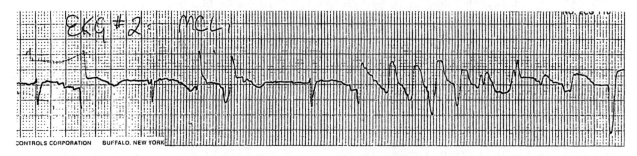

FIGURE 12.2

I decided I didn't like the looks of those runs of V tach, so I whacked him in the chest. The runs of V tach stopped. Mr. McDougal woke up. I debated with myself about giving him some lidocaine, getting him on oxygen, and the like. But we were right there at the hospital door, and I didn't see the benefit of staying in the ambulance any longer. So we quickly wheeled him into an emergency room that wasn't expecting anything more than another nonemergent patient.

I quickly told Mr. McDougal's story, explained what I had done and why I had done it, and reported his brief seizure and cardiac arrest on our arrival. For some reason (I believe the nurse was preoccupied with two other critical patients at the time), my message didn't get across. The nurse picked up on the emotional hyperventilation aspects and tried to direct us to a back room that was barely equipped with a cardiac monitor. While I was trying to explain that he needed lidocaine and a critical care room, Mr. McDougal seized again.

By the time he was in a critical care room and back on a monitor, Mr. McDougal was in ventricular fibrillation. He was successfully defibrillated and finally got some lidocaine. The reason for his arrest became apparent once his lab values were determined. His potassium level was 2.0. The normal potassium level ranges from 3.5 to 5.0.

There are several standard clues to suspecting hypokalemia in a patient. Diuretic use is the classic clue. People on Lasix, hydrochlorothiazide, and the like, who don't have (or don't take) a potassium supplement, are prone to hypokalemia. Mr. McDougal wasn't on a diuretic, but his excessive water intake probably produced a hypotonic overhydration that diluted his electrolytes, specifically his potassium. The classic EKG finding for a patient with hypokalemia is flattened T waves with prominent U waves.

Although I hadn't recognized that Mr. McDougal's "prolonged QT segments" were actually flat T waves with prominent U waves, I had at least recognized the indications of a potential electrolyte disturbance and started an IV. As I continued to reflect on the call, I became a little pale and sweaty myself. If Mr. McDougal's apartment hadn't been such a mess, if he had "only" been mugged, humiliated, and frightened by his wife's hang-up, I probably would have left him at home. This was a case where burglary and a ransacked apartment had saved someone's life!

Our next case study involves a 14-year-old boy named Jimmy. Jimmy was out skateboarding with some friends, came home, climbed to his third-floor apartment and said, "Mom, I don't feel…" and collapsed to the floor in mid-sentence. No one in this particular apartment building had a phone, so someone ran a block and a half to a pay phone to call 911. When we arrived, our first responders were treating Jimmy with nasal cannula oxygen. Unfortunately, Jimmy was in cardiopulmonary arrest. We initiated CPR and Figure 12.3 is Jimmy's quick look.

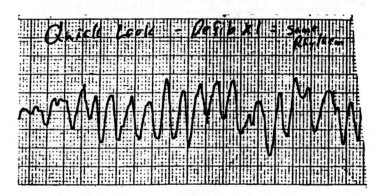

FIGURE 12.3

We defibrillated that a few times, without effect. This call occurred back in the days when sodium bicarb was one of the first medications you administered in an arrest with a long "down time," so we gave Jimmy an amp of bicarb, 75 milligrams of lidocaine, 250 milligrams of Bretylium, and defibrillated him again. Figure 12.4 was what resulted from that treatment.

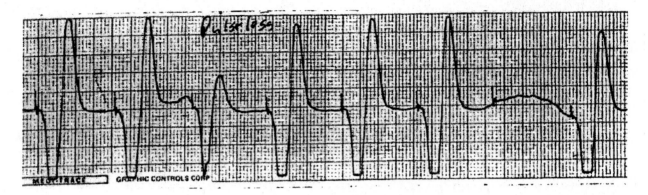

FIGURE 12.4

This EKG strip may look familiar to you. It's the same strip as that of Figure 10.5. This is a paced rhythm with occasionally ineffective capture. Unfortunately, it was also pulseless. So we continued CPR and began following the EMD (now called "PEA") protocols by administering a fluid challenge as we extricated Jimmy from the third floor. Back in those days we also used MAST pants for EMD. We got to the ambulance, put on the MAST pants, blew them up, and Jimmy quickly converted to the rhythm you see in Figure 12.5.

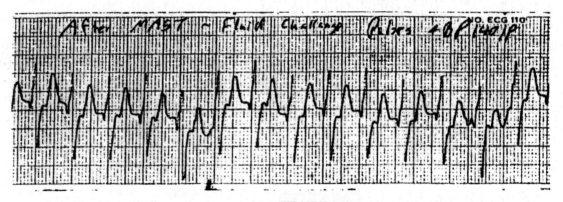

FIGURE 12.5

With this rhythm, Jimmy had pulses and a systolic blood pressure of 140. By now I'm sure you're wondering, "Why does a 14-year-old boy have a pacemaker?!" I'll tell you why. Jimmy had a history of sick sinus syndrome. I don't have a copy of his EKG prior to receiving a pacemaker, but I do have an example of what it might have looked like. With this example, we'll briefly divert to another case, but come right back to Jimmy.

Figure 12.6 is the EKG of a 37-year-old male who had a chief complaint of "vertigo." He didn't call it dizziness, he called it vertigo, and he had no other associated complaints. Figure 12.6 is a classic example of sick sinus syndrome. It shows episodes of tachycardia alternating with episodes of bradycardia. (In this particular EKG there are other things going on besides a sick sinus, but the sick sinus certainly would explain the complaint of "vertigo.")

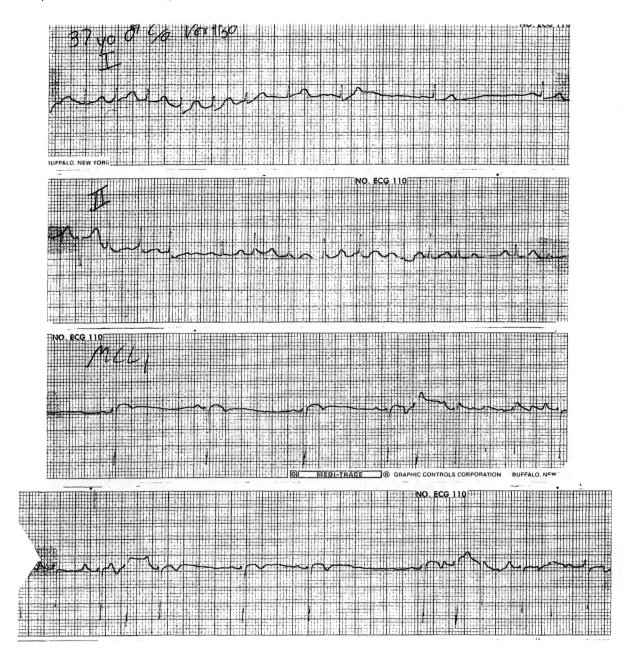

FIGURE 12.6

How do you suppose a sick sinus syndrome is treated? Of course you've been clued into the use of a pacemaker. But a pacemaker will only take care of the bradycardia episodes. In addition to their pacemaker, these patients need medication to control their tachycardias. Usually, their private physician will experiment with several medications before finding one that has an optimal effect. Sometimes it may be a slow-channel calcium blocker, such as verapamil. Sometimes a beta-blocking medication, such as Tenormin or Lopressor, works out better. And, sometimes, digitalis ends up being the optimal medication.

In Jimmy's case, digitalis was the drug of choice to treat the tachycardia caused by his sick sinus syndrome. Unfortunately, what some physicians don't remember is that digitalis is also a mild diuretic. You can lose potassium when taking it. Jimmy's physician put in a pacemaker, medicated him with digitalis, but forgot to tell Jimmy to eat a banana every day.

The cause of Jimmy's arrest, as with Mr. McDougal's arrest, was hypokalemia. Jimmy's potassium level was 2.8. Happily, Jimmy was an otherwise healthy young boy who walked out of the hospital a few days later with no deficits from his close experience with death. And I'm sure no one needed to remind him to eat his bananas after that.

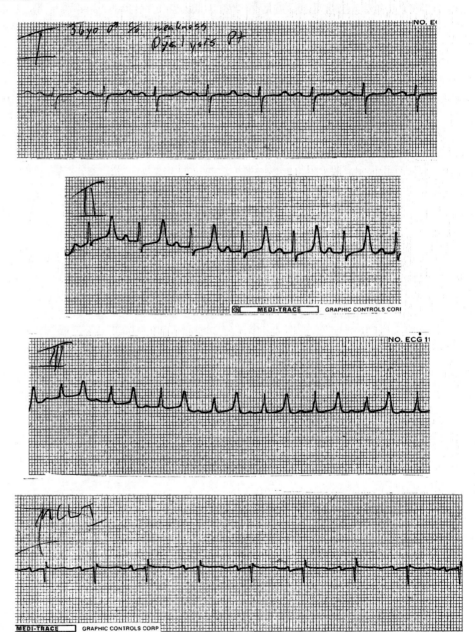

FIGURE 12.7

I'm not going to present an in-depth case study for Figure 12.7. But I include this EKG to round out the previous two patient cases with a *hyper-kalemic* strip and some discussion of hyperkalemia. Do you remember the Mike Taigman Rule of Hyperkalemic T Waves from Chapter One? When the T waves look like they would hurt your butt if you sat on them, the patient is probably hyperkalemic. Hyperkalemia is not limited to T wave changes, however. The amount of EKG changes increases as the patient's potassium level rises. Some of the widest QRS complexes I've ever seen were those of hyperkalemic patients.

Before you can appreciate changes on the electrocardiogram, however, you need to ensure a correctly calibrated EKG monitor. If you don't already calibrate your monitor at the beginning of *each* EKG, you should. The calibration box should measure 10 millivolts (two large boxes tall). Without standard calibration of the prehospital EKG, it's difficult to accurately diagnose things like hyperkalemia, and comparisons cannot be made with the patient's 12 lead later at the hospital.

Now, back to hyperkalemia. What group of patients are most likely to have episodes of hyperkalemia? Dialysis patients. Figure 12.7 is the EKG of a 36-year-old male dialysis patient. Dialysis patients may become hyperkalemic when overdue for dialysis (having missed one or more treatments) or when they are experiencing an increase in their renal failure. Another group of patients susceptible to hyperkalemia may surprise you: people taking herbal vitamin and mineral supplements. Normal use of these supplements is quite healthy and unharmful. Unfortunately, some people feel the need to take megadoses of the stuff. These people may accidently overdose themselves on potassium.

Alterations in other electrolyte levels can also affect the electrocardiogram. Calcium plays a very important role in cardiac electrical activity. Hypocalcemic patients develop long Q-T intervals (Figure 12.8). The Q-T interval is measured from the beginning of the QRS complex to the end of the T wave.

Within normal rates (between 60 to 110 beats per minute), the Q-T interval should be less than half the distance of the previous R-R measurement. If there is a significant bradycardia or tachycardia present, however, there is a correction factor that must be considered. I've included a Normal Q-T Interval table to give you an idea of how the Q-T interval is normally altered by changes in rates.

Normal Q-T Intervals

Heart Rate per Minute	Men and Children (seconds)	Women (seconds)
40	0.449–0.491	0.461–0.503
50	0.414–0.413	0.425–0.464
60	0.386–0.422	0.396–0.432
70.5	0.361–0.395	0.371–0.405
80	0.342–0.374	0.352–0.384
92.5	0.321–0.351	0.330–0.360
100	0.310–0.338	0.318–0.347
109	0.297–0.325	0.305–0.333
120	0.283–0.310	0.291–0.317
133	0.268–0.294	0.276–0.301
150	0.252–0.275	0.258–0.282
172	0.234–0.255	0.240–0.262

Adapted from the table "Normal Q-T Intervals and the Upper Limits of the Normal," from R. Ashman and E. Hull, *Essentials of Electrocardiography*, Macmillan Company, New York, 1945.

As you can see from the measurements listed, the Q-T interval normally becomes longer as the rate becomes slower and shorter as the rate becomes faster. If you don't routinely carry a "Normal Q-T Intervals" chart with you, simply remember this: bradycardias may normally have long Q-T intervals, and tachycardias may have short Q-T intervals; but within normal rates (60 to 110), the Q-T interval should be half the distance of the preceding R-R interval. If it is longer, suspect hypocalcemia.

Q-T Interval Norms

Bradycardias may normally have long Q-T intervals. Tachycardias may have short Q-T intervals.

But within normal rates (60 to 110), the Q-T interval should be half the distance of the preceding R-R interval.

If it is longer, suspect hypocalcemia.

What kind of patients are likely to have hypocalcemia? Patients who have a hypothyroid condition or patients who have had their thyroid *and parathyroids* removed. Twelve or more years ago, surgeons thought that the parathyroid glands were just little globules of fat and routinely cut them out along with the thyroid when doing thyroidectomies. Since then, they have learned what the parathyroid glands are and how important they are for mediating calcium. If persons without parathyroid glands aren't taking calcium supplements on a regular basis, they can easily become hypocalcemic.

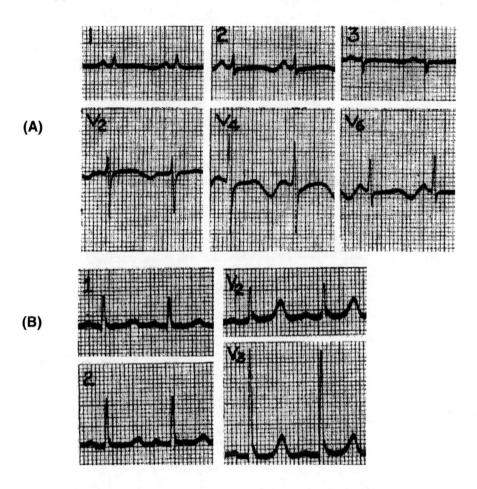

FIGURE 12.8 (A) **Hypocalcemia**. Note the prolonged Q–T interval in an otherwise normal tracing. Q–T = 0.40 sec (upper limit of normal for this rate and sex is 0.35 sec). Patient's serum calcium was 7.0 mg per 100 ml, other electrolytes being normal. (B) **Hypocalcemia**. Note prolonged ST and QT with late inversion of T waves. From a patient with serum calcium of 4.2 mg per 100 ml. (Henry J. L., Marriott: *Practical Electrocardiography*, 8th ed., 1988; Williams & Wilkins, Baltimore.)

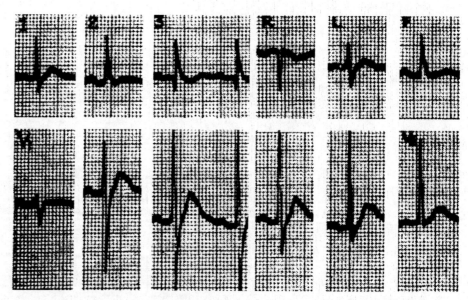

FIGURE 12.9 (Henry J. L. Marriott: *Practical Electrocardiography*, 8th ed., 1988; Williams & Wilkins, Baltimore.)

Usually, the chief complaint of someone who has become hypocalcemic is abdominal or chest "cramps." Their initial complaints are similar to those voiced by people who have been bitten by a black widow spider. Somehow, the poison of a black widow spider bite produces reduced calcium levels (thus the reason for administration of calcium to victims of black widow spider bites). Tetany and tetanus occur due to the same process.

As for *hyper*calcemia, it shortens the Q-T interval (Figure 12.9). In some cases, the Q-T interval becomes so short that it appears to be an elevated S-T segment, or you might even think it was a J wave (Osborne wave) caused by hypothermia. Of course, if your patient was just extricated from a frozen-meat locker, it's certainly more likely that you are looking at J waves. But if there is no history of hypothermic exposure, this finding would indicate hypercalcemia. Hypercalcemic patients are usually those who overdose on calcium supplements.

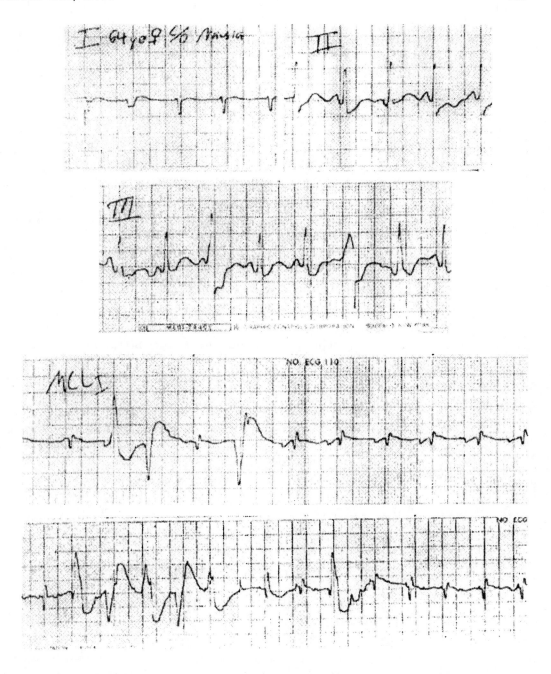

FIGURE 12.10

Mrs. Fowler, a 64-year-old female, called 911 complaining of nausea "all day long." Figure 12.10 is her prehospital electrocardiogram. I think you can see why Mrs. Fowler was having nausea. She has a slight sinus tachycardia and a right axis deviation. What does that indicate? Right! A left posterior hemiblock. Her wide QRSs are multifocal, but are most appropriately called bidirectional. She has periods of alternating left and right ventricular tachycardia. Hence, her ectopy occurs from both directions and is called *bidirectional ventricular tachycardia.*

Bidirectional ventricular tachycardia is frequently diagnostic of digitalis toxicity. Digitalis (often called *dig*, and pronounced "didge") is a great drug. But keep in mind what a cardiologist once told me about *dig*: "If you've got a patient with a bizarre EKG and she's *not* on digitalis, she probably should be. And if you've got a patient with a bizarre EKG and she's *on* digitalis, she is probably on too much of it."

Mrs. Fowler was seriously "*dig* toxic." One of the first symptoms of almost any toxicity is nausea. Classically, patients who are *dig* toxic describe halos around lights and objects. If you have seen the painting by Vincent Van Gogh entitled "Starry Night," you have seen what the world looks like to a *dig* toxic patient. Later in his life, Van Gogh developed an irregular heart condition and was eating foxglove leaves and drinking foxglove tea for it. Foxglove is the original vegetable source for digitalis. When he painted "Starry Night," Van Gogh was probably *dig* toxic and was seeing halos around everything. His later paintings reflect this with the sweeping, circular paint strokes that create halos around his subjects. So, along with bidirectional ventricular tachycardia, a patient's description of halo hallucinations should immediately make you suspicious of digitalis toxicity.

Figure 12.11 is the next in my presentation of wild and crazy EKGs. I don't have an MCL$_1$ strip, but using the leads available, what would you call this EKG? Well, it's hard to say. There are clearly some occasional dropped beats that produce groups of beats. The P-R intervals are relatively constant and within normal limits, but there is at least one incident of what looks like A-V dissociation. The R-R intervals don't progressively shorten, and twice the shortest R-R interval is not necessarily longer than the longest R-R interval. The QRS complexes are within normal limits, so there is no bundle branch block. This EKG just doesn't seem to want to fit any single set of rules!

When that happens, and it sometimes will, take a break and look at something else. Is there an infarction going on? Yes. As stated in Chapter Eleven, the indicative changes (S-T elevation) you see in leads II and III, paired with the *reciprocal* changes (S-T depression) in lead I, indicate an inferior infarction occurring. Does that assist you in diagnosing the underlying rhythm? In this case it does. The occasional dropped beats A-V heart block that is most often associated with inferior infarctions is occasional dropped beats type I, or Wenckebach.

Figure 12.11 is a Wenckebach. I'll admit it's a very unusual Wenckebach and may have some occasional junctional escape beats overriding some of the P waves. But, I needed to use this strip to call your attention to a specific variety of S-T segment. If you wanted to "paint a picture" of this EKG on the phone or radio, what could you say about the S-T segments?

These are called "tombstone S-T segments." Not only do they look like the old-style, rounded tombstones, there is plenty of room for you to write an appropriate epitaph within the T waves. The appearance of tombstone S-T segments is a true predictor of the outcome for the patient who has this sort of EKG finding. They often die.

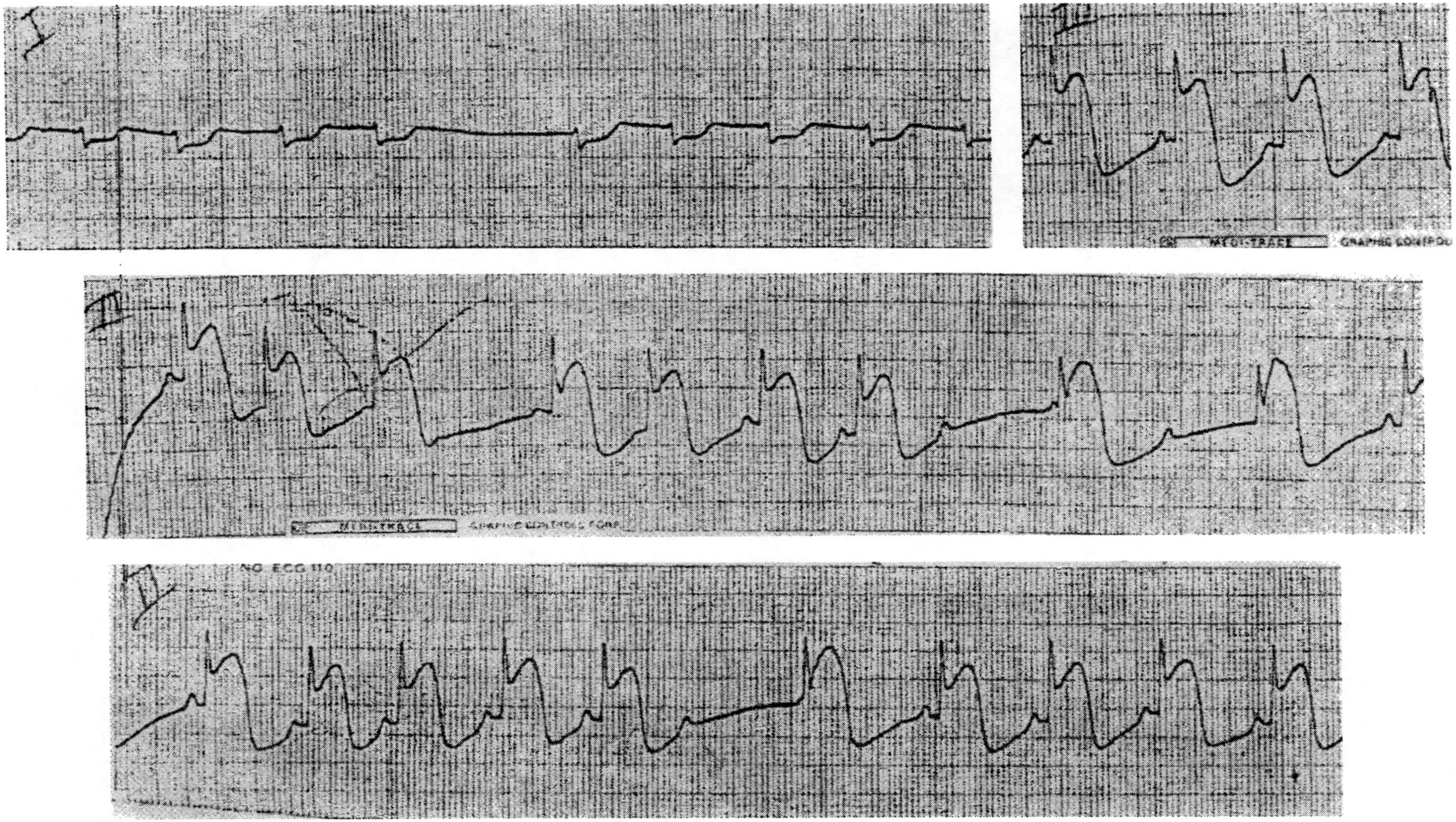

FIGURE 12.11

Figure 12.12 is the EKG of a 59-year-old female with a gunshot wound to the head. She had been lying outdoors, unconscious, for approximately 24 hours, so she was also hypothermic. In fact, her core temperature was 87 degrees Fahrenheit. Unfortunately, I only have her lead II strip. I include this strip to introduce another descriptive term for EKG reporting: *cerebral T waves.*

Increased intercranial pressure (ICP), whether from a CVA or a traumatic head injury, often produces this type of T wave inversion. Thus, they are called cerebral T waves. They are smooth, dipping T waves that look as though someone hooked their finger over the S-T segment and pulled the T wave down. Because this particular patient was also hypothermic, there is a J wave prior to each cerebral T wave.

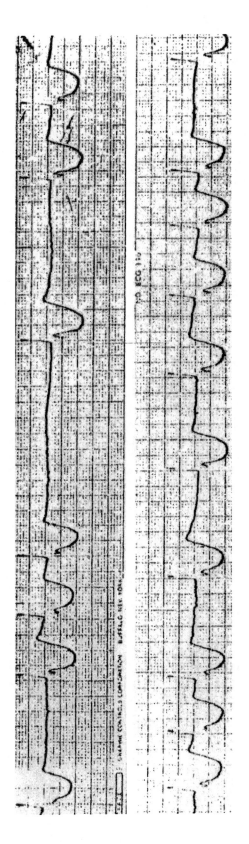

FIGURE 12.12

Eighty-three year-old Mrs. Carpenter had chest pain and called 911. Figure 12.13 is the initial EKG seen by the responding paramedics. As their interview continued, suddenly Mrs. Carpenter stopped talking to them and appeared to have some fine seizure activity. When they glanced at the monitor, Figure 12.14 is what they saw.

Seeing this strip, the responders initiated CPR. Whereupon Mrs. Carpenter pushed them off her chest and yelled, "That hurts! Stop it!" Naturally, Mrs. Carpenter's responders were surprised and a little confused by her response. Her EKG had resumed the rhythm of Figure 12.13 and they decided to "cut and run." She received oxygen, an IV line, and an accelerator—their vehicle's accelerator.

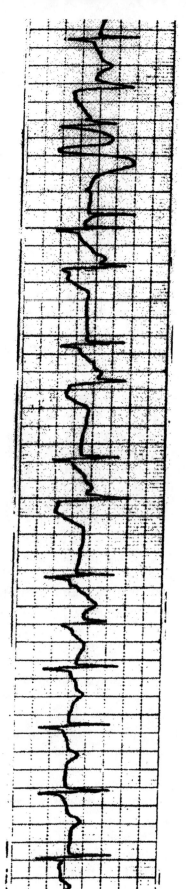

FIGURE 12.13

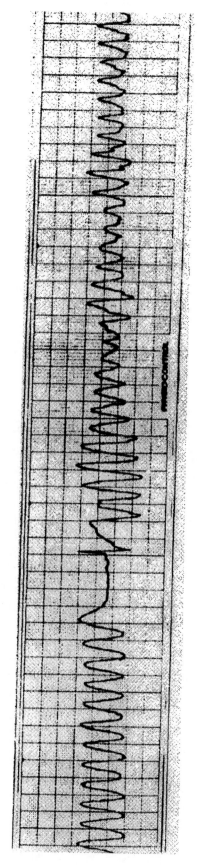

FIGURE 12.14

203

In spite of everything, Mrs. Carpenter survived to arrive at the hospital. Figure 12.15 is her 12-lead EKG. Look at the extended lead II strip along the bottom of her 12 lead. Measure her Q-T intervals, remembering the general guideline for normal Q-T intervals: within normal rates (between 60 to 110 beats per minute), the Q-T interval should be less than half the distance of the previous R-R measurement. Mrs. Carpenter's average R-R interval is 0.72 seconds. Half of that is 0.36 seconds, but her average Q-T interval is about 0.48 seconds. Mrs. Carpenter had considerably prolonged Q-T intervals. Q-T interval prolongation is one of the few known predictive factors for the development of *torsade de pointes*. In Figure 12.14, Mrs. Carpenter was in torsade de pointes.

Some literature references spell the term *torsades* de pointes, others *torsade* de pointes. I prefer the latter but will usually refer to it, simply as torsades. Several different terms have been used to describe torsades, such as paroxysmal ventricular fibrillation, atypical ventricular tachycardia, and polymorphous or multifocal ventricular tachycardia. The most accurate description is probably *multifocal ventricular tachycardia.*

Torsade de pointes is French for "torsion of the points," a phrase that reflects the twisting morphology created by polarity changes of the QRS complexes. The points of the QRS complexes rhythmically change from positive to negative, twisting or squeezing together as the polarity changes back and forth. Thus, there are QRS complexes pointing downward, twisting and becoming smaller as the polarity changes, then pointing upward, then twisting and becoming smaller, then downward, and so on. The classic appearance created by this phenomenon is one of repeating "bow ties" of V tach.

Often, one or more normal QRS complexes will be interspersed between the bow-tie twists of torsades, and patients may spontaneously convert to their previous underlying rhythm. Or they may go the other way and completely degenerate into ventricular fibrillation. Marriott considers torsade de pointes as being an intermediary point between ventricular tachycardia and ventricular fibrillation.

The mechanism of torsade de pointes is probably a form of reentry,[1] or it may result from mutual competition of ectopic sites in each ventricle.[2] Basically, researchers haven't been able to firmly and consistently support any specific mechanism as yet. The only thing they do agree on is that torsade de pointes is frequently associated with prolonged Q-T intervals.

Q-T intervals can be prolonged by physiological or pharmacological causes. Physiological causes include intrinsic myocardial disease, brady dysrhythmias, liquid protein diets, electrolyte disturbances, organophosphate poisoning, and closed head injuries. Medications that prolong the Q-T interval include phenothiazines[3] and a multitude of antidysrhythmics: procainamide (Pronestyl, Procan), disopyramide (Norpace), flecainide (Tambocor), encainide (Enkaid),[*] and amiodarone (Cordarone).[4] A few calcium channel blockers, for example, bepridil (Vascor) and nicardipine (Cardene), are known to prolong the Q-T interval.[5] The beta blocker

---

*Encainide (Enkaid) has been voluntarily withdrawn from the market by the manufacturer but remains available on a limited basis.

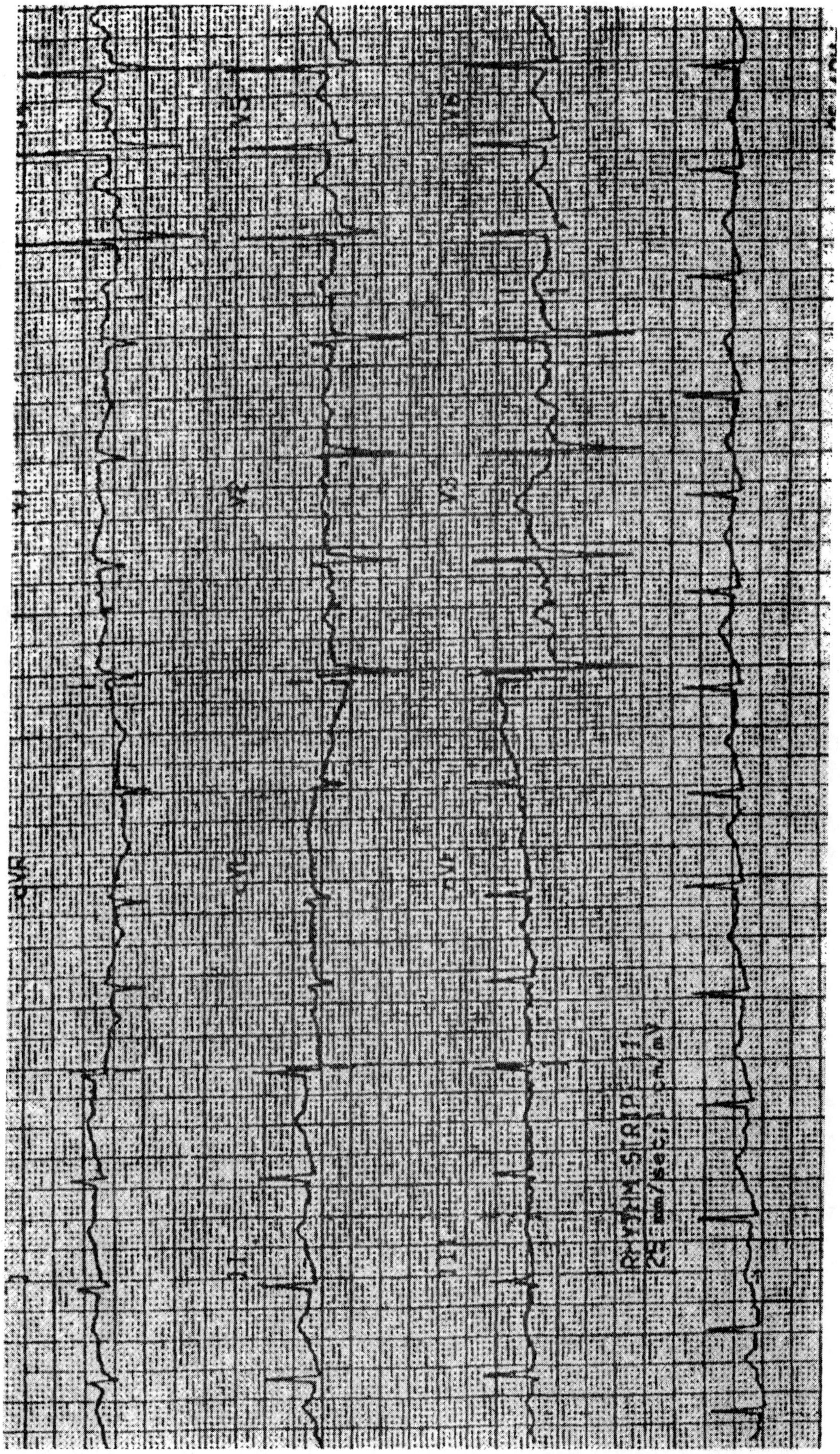

FIGURE 12.15

sotalol (Betapace) is notorious for prolonging Q-T intervals.[6] But the anti-dysrhythmics most easily remembered as causing Q-T interval prolongation are the quinidine family; Quinora, Quinidex, Quinaglute, Quinalan, and Cardioquin.[7,8,9] Mrs. Carpenter (Figures 12.13, 12.14 and 12.15) had a history of premature atrial ectopy and was being treated with quinidine.

Torsade de pointes is a ventricular tachyarrhythmia that is frequently refractory to conventional treatment.[9] Torsades often resists cardioversion or defibrillation. Surprisingly, it appears to respond well to precordial thump conversion, however, the conversion may be transient and repeated thumps may be required.[10] In Mrs. Carpenter's case, the initiation of CPR was her "precordial thump," and the conversion lasted to the hospital.

Because its underlying etiology is a prolonged Q-T interval, torsade de pointes is often considered a contraindication to the administration of lidocaine.[9,10] Lidocaine is known to prolong Q-T intervals. (In spite of this, lidocaine has also occasionally appeared successful in the conversion of torsades.)

Because of their ability to shorten ventricular refractory times, *atropine* and *Isuprel* were once the time-honored drugs of choice for Torsades treatment.[7,9] (Can you picture yourself calling in for orders to administer *atropine* or *Isuprel* to a patient in "ventricular tachycardia"?!) Recommended treatments now include overdrive pacing and/or magnesium sulphate.[11]

Hypomagnesemia (along with hypocalcemia and hypokalemia) is considered an electrolyte disturbance productive of long Q-T intervals—and thus productive of torsade de pointes. Yet magnesium sulphate has been found to effectively treat Torsades even in the presence of *normal* plasma magnesium levels.[11] Magnesium sulphate does not shorten Q-T intervals. At this writing, researchers aren't quite sure *why* it works for Torsades.

Other medications successfully used to convert Torsades include phenytoin and bretylium.[9,11, 12] All in all, torsades de pointes is an interesting and challenging arrhythmia. Continued research will undoubtedly produce an even better understanding of the Torsades phenomenon and lead to more definitive and well-understood methods of treatment.

Larry is our next case study. Larry was a 24-year-old male who had just graduated from military basic training. Naturally, he celebrated his freedom from forced abstention by imbibing an incredible quantity of an equally impressive variety of alcoholic beverages. Larry awoke the following morning alone, in an unfamiliar car, in a neighborhood he didn't recognize, with chest pain. He described "crushing," substernal chest pain, radiating to the left side of his neck and down his left arm. He was pale, cool, diaphoretic. He was short of breath. And—oh yeah—Larry also had a headache and a good deal of nausea.

The paramedic who responded to attend to Larry found it difficult to attribute his complaints to an acute myocardial infarction because of his age and general history. He appeared physically fit, didn't smoke, didn't chronically abuse alcohol, had no family history of cardiac disease, and he was a 24-year-old male. When she ran an EKG on Larry, Figure 12.16 is what the paramedic saw.

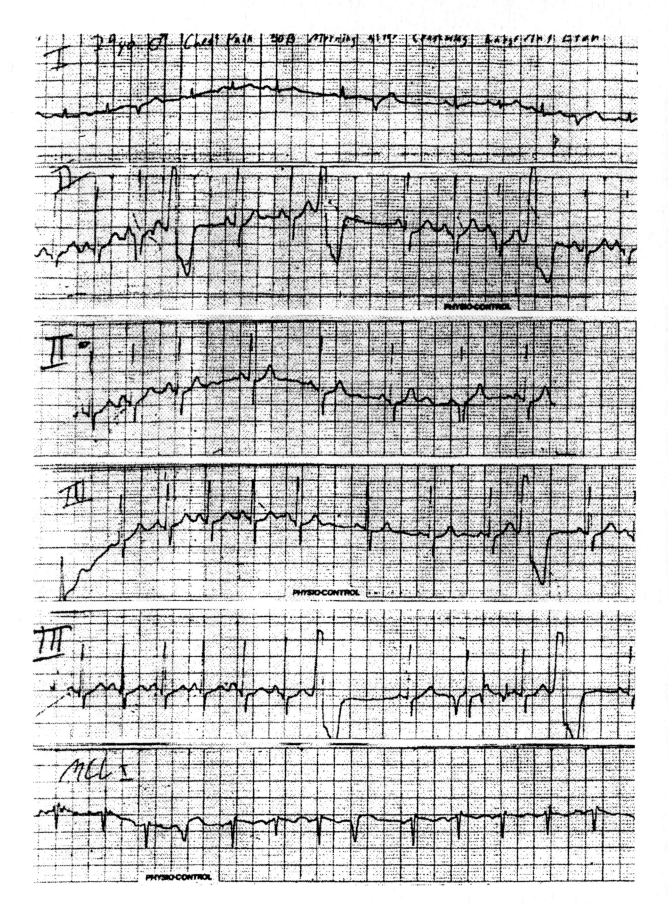

FIGURE 12.16

He had an irregularly irregular rhythm, normal axis, sinus tachycardia with periods of wandering atrial pacemaker, and frequent, unifocal PVCs. The paramedic wisely decided to ignore his young age and pristine health history. She treated Larry for an acute myocardial infarction.

"Holiday heart syndrome" occurs when an acute ingestion of large amounts of ethanol causes an irritation of the myocardium and/or a coronary artery spasm. This may produce any of the complaints and dysrhythmias associated with acute myocardial infarction. Atrial fibrillation, atrial flutter, and wandering atrial pacemaker are common manifestations of holiday heart syndrome. Youth and exceptional good health do not protect a person from this syndrome, but usually provide for a better prognosis than would be anticipated in an older, less fit person.

Since holiday heart syndrome does not involve an occlusion of plaque or clots, thrombolytic drugs are unnecessary. If a sufficient amount of collateral circulation is present, and the patient survives the arrhythmias, holiday heart syndrome rarely results in myocardial necrosis. It simply requires supportive management and time to naturally resolve the alcohol poisoning.

The greatest danger of this syndrome is the propensity of all types of health care providers (including MDs) to casually attribute a young, healthy person's infarctionlike complaints to a "high porcelain content" (a term derived from hugging the toilet after drinking too much). Consequently, patients may receive only rehydration and dextrose. Without aggressive support and appropriate ACLS management, however, these young healthy patients may progress to a permanent infarction—and even death.

And now, our last case presentation. Several years ago, on a sunny afternoon, my partner and I were dispatched on a "sick case, nausea/vomiting" call. Because of the seemingly simple call nature and affluent location, our dispatchers anticipated no need for fire department or police assistance. Just I and my partner responded.

On arrival, we noted that our patient lived in a lovely apartment building on the fourth floor. We subsequently discovered that the building had only one elevator, and it was out of service. After lugging our equipment up eight, winding half-flights of stairs, we finally arrived at the patient's apartment.

The patient's wife let us into the apartment and led us to the kitchen, telling us that "George" had been vomiting "all day long" and had suffered a syncopal episode just moments before our arrival. She reported he was 54 years old, adding, "This happened to him once before, and he almost died!"

When we reached the kitchen, the first thing I noticed was that George was a rather large gentleman and was crawling around on the floor in a very agitated manner. But what really impressed me was how pasty-white and sweaty he was. George was drenched in sweat to the point where it looked like he'd just crawled out of the shower.

We quickly laid him flat on his couch and proceeded with our exam. He had a respiratory rate of 40 and was not able to communicate effectively at all. His weak radial pulse was too rapid for me to count easily, but I was able to palpate a systolic blood pressure of 62. (Don't you find it funny that the presence of a radial pulse is supposed to indicate a systolic blood pressure of at least 80, but you can palpate blood pressures of only 60? I do.)

As my partner applied the monitor patches, I questioned George's wife. She reported that George's only complaints had been nausea and vomiting. There was no blood in his emesis—just bile-colored fluid. He never mentioned chest pain, shortness of breath, or abdominal pain and had no recent illness or trauma. She assured us that he was compliant with his medication, which was Lanoxin (a digitalis derivative). Figure 12.17 is the electrocardiogram we obtained.

Figure 12.17 shows a regular tachycardia, at a rate of about 200 to 220 beats per minute, that may or may not have wide QRS complexes. There is a left axis deviation—that's not diagnostically helpful. There are occasional blips that may or may not be P waves—they aren't consistent enough to map out, though. The QRS complex morphology in leads MCL_1 and MCL_6 is unhelpful, and there is no concordancy between them—that's also unhelpful.

My partner and I disagreed about whether this EKG was supraventricular or ventricular. He believed that this patient was in supraventricular tachycardia with left bundle branch block aberration. When asked to explain his opinion, he didn't cite any morphological criteria or statistical analysis. He simply said, "It *looks* like supraventricular tachycardia."

I was more scientific. I *analyzed* the rhythm! Although I couldn't find morphological support in MCL_1 or MCL_6 for V tach, I decided George had very wide QRS complexes (about 0.16 seconds wide). Complexes of that width most often favor ventricular tachycardia. And, in the end, it came down to my old rule for wide complex tachycardias: if you don't have a good reason to diagnose supraventricular tachycardia, treat it like V tach.

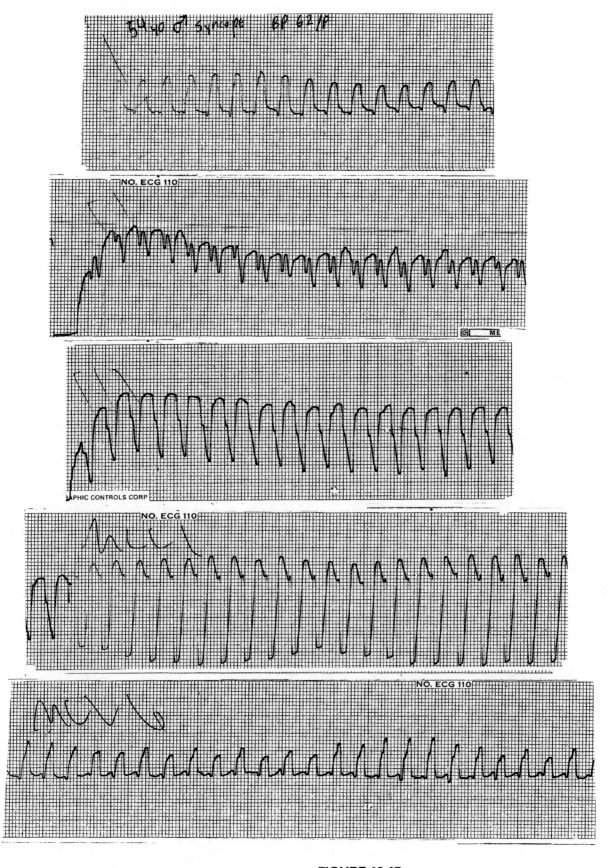

FIGURE 12.17

So, since I was the patient attendant that shift, we did. After calling for the fire department's help (remembering that we were going to have to get rather-large-George down eight skinny flights of stairs), we started an IV and gave him some lidocaine. It didn't help. After that I called my medical control physician (lets call him Dr. Zed) to discuss cardioversion and administration of Valium. My request was denied. Like many other physicians, Dr. Zed was rather hesitant to order cardioversion for a digital-ized patient with a tachycardia, even though it was "symptomatic." People who are on digitalis and have tachycardias often cardiovert to asystole—and stay there. So even though George was hypotensive, we were ordered to try bretylium. We administered a bretylium drip. It made George want to vomit all the more, increased his agitation, and didn't change his tachy-cardia. When we called him back, Dr. Zed suggested we make an emer-gency run to the closest hospital.

So we carried this sweaty, agitated, hypoperfusing patient down eight flights of stairs and applied our trusty vehicle accelerator. Despite my defibrillation paddles gelled and ready, George managed to persist in his tachycardia throughout the trip to the hospital without progressing to ventricular fibrillation.

At the hospital, the receiving physician also knew to avoid cardiovert-ing a patient with digitalized tachycardia. He decided to attempt it anyway. But he wanted to make sure that—whatever the rhythm was—it converted on the first shot, so he ordered the patient to be cardioverted at 300 watt-seconds. George's chest ended up "medium well," but his tachycardia imme-diately converted to a sinus rhythm—a sinus rhythm with QRS complexes with exactly the same width and deflections of those seen in Figure 12.17.

George's rhythm had, in fact, been a supraventricular tachycardia. But there was no way that I or the emergency room could diagnose that from his EKG. The bottom line is this: even when you've studied a lot about EKGs, there are exceptions to every rule you'll ever learn. When it comes to playing with wide complex tachycardias, you're playing the percentages. And sometimes the percentages are wrong.

That concludes our "Wild and Crazy EKGs" chapter. I hope you've enjoyed (and profited from) these cases as much as I have. One of the most magical and motivating aspects of our profession is that we never, ever stop learning. Just when we begin to think that we've seen or done it all, there's always a new study or a different twist of events to fire us up again.

REFERENCES

1. Horowitz, L. N.: Torsades de pointes; electrophysiologic studies in patients with transient pharmacologic or metabolic abnormalities. *Circulation* 1981:63, 1120.

2. D'Alnoncourt, C. N., et al. Torsade de pointes tachycardia: Re-entry or focal activity? *Br Heart J* 1982; 48:213.

3. *Drug Facts and Comparisons*, J. B. Lippincott Co., St. Louis, MO: 1990; p. 265f (phenothiazines).

4. *Drug Facts and Comparisons,* J. B. Lippincott Co., St. Louis, MO: 1992; pp. 145k (procainamide), 146b (disopyramide), 148c (flecainide), 147h (encainide), 148l (amiodarone).

5. *Drug Facts and Comparisons,* J. B. Lippincott Co., St. Louis, MO: 1992; pp. 149c (bepridil), 149n (nicardipine).

6. *Drug Facts and Comparisons,* J. B. Lippincott Co., St. Louis, MO: 1993; p. 158r (sotalol).

7. Morrison, Y., and Thompson, D.F.: Isoproterenol treatment of torsades de pointes. *Ann Pharmacother,* 1993; 27(2):189–90.

8. *Drug Facts and Comparisons,* J. B. Lippincott Co., St. Louis, MO: 1992; p. 145c (quinidine).

9. Vukmir, R.B.: Torsades de pointes: a review. *Am J Emerg Med,* 1991; 9(3):250–5.

10. Taigman M. and Canan S: Cardiology practicum; torsade de pointes. *JEMS,* Feb. 1987, pp. 48–9.

11. Napolitano, C., Priori, S. G., Schwartz, P. J.: Torsade de pointes, mechanisms and management. *Drugs,* Jan. 1994, pp. 51–65.

12. Martinez, R.: Torsades de pointes: atypical rhythm, atypical treatment. *Ann Emerg Med,* 1987; 16(8):878–84.

CHAPTER 13

Practice EKG Strips and Text Summary

To complete this text, I have assembled a variety of practice EKG strips. Most of these strips are presented with case study information. Some are simply for exercising your new diagnostic skills. On the flip side of each strip presentation, you will find my interpretation of the EKG.

Remember to develop your own standard approach to electrocardiogram interpretation. As in Chapter Five, my suggestion is to first look at the QRS rate; is it fast, slow, or within normal limits (WNL)? Then look at any patterns of regularity or irregularity. Are there groups of beats? Then look at the axis. Does the axis indicate the presence of a hemiblock? Once the axis is determined, look at the width of the QRS complexes. Are they within normal limits? If they are wide, are they originating in the ventricles or is there a bundle branch blocked (BBB)? If a BBB is present, which one is it? Then observe the P waves (are there any?) and their relationship to the QRS complexes (do they have one and, if so, how long is the P-R interval?). After that you can identify arrhythmias, ectopy, infarction patterns—all that other stuff!

Refer to the appendix if you need to look at Chapter Eight's algorithm for differentiating V tach from SVT with aberration, or the morphological clues suggestive of V tach, or Chapter Eleven's patterns of changes often seen accompanying myocardial infarctions.

Taigman's Standard Approach to EKGs

1. QRS rate; fast, slow, or within normal limits (WNL)?

2. Is it regular or irregular? *Groups* of beats?

3. What is the axis? Is there a hemiblock?

4. Width of the QRS complexes: WNL or BBB? (Left or Right BBB?)

5. P waves. Are there any? Are they related to the QRS complexes? If so, what is the P-R interval?

6. Is an arrhythmia present?

7. Is ectopy present?

8. Is an infarction present?

CASE NUMBER ONE:

We were called to the residence of a 62-year-old female because of a possible psychiatric emergency. We found her sitting on the floor, ranting and raving incoherently. Her family members were convinced that she had gone off the deep end. A quick check of her radial pulse revealed that one could barely be felt. Her carotid pulse was rapid and weak. Her blood pressure was 68 by palpation. Her respiratory rate was 34 and shallow. She was pale, she was cool, she was diaphoretic, and she was very confused. Figure 13.1 is her EKG.

This EKG shows leads I, II, III, MCL_1, and MCL_6 of a wide complex tachycardia. Her family could provide no significant medical history. They knew nothing about her medications, allergies, or anything that preceded her deterioration.

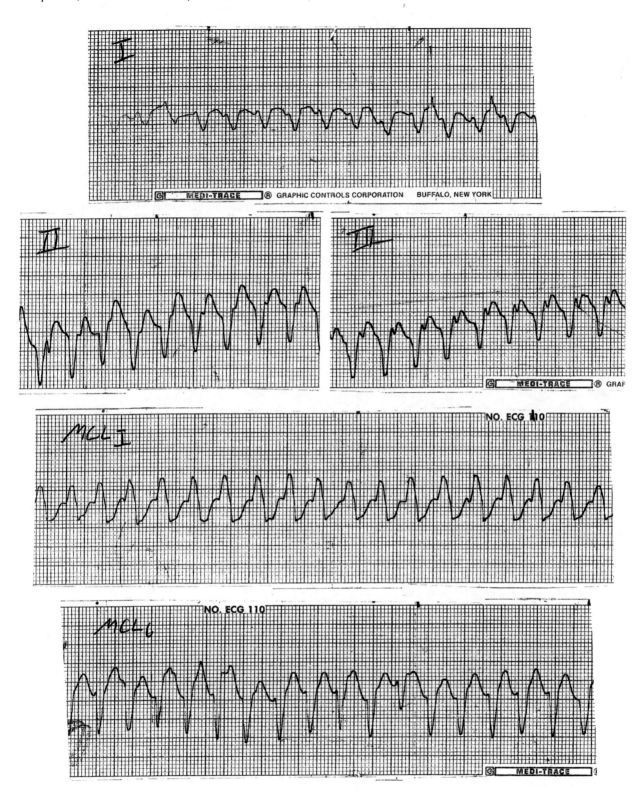

FIGURE 13.1

This patient is obviously hypoperfusing and something needs to be done to restore her level of consciousness and blood pressure. Observation of leads I, II, and III reveals a right shoulder axis (negative QRS complexes in each of those leads). She has a wide complex tachycardia. Looking at MCL$_1$, you see an upright complex with a left rabbit ear taller than the right. It's not a clear rabbit ear, it's more of a slur. But that still is strongly supportive of ventricular tachycardia. She also has a little r and deep wide S complex in MCL$_6$. Again, this is strongly supportive of ventricular tachycardia. Combined with the right shoulder axis (itself favoring ventricular tachycardia), these morphological clues clearly indicate that this patient should be treated for ventricular tachycardia.

There is some debate as to whether this patient should be managed electrically or chemically. We elected to start an IV line and administer a bolus of lidocaine, which successfully converted her rhythm. This patient's underlying problem was an acute myocardial infarction. She ended up doing just fine.

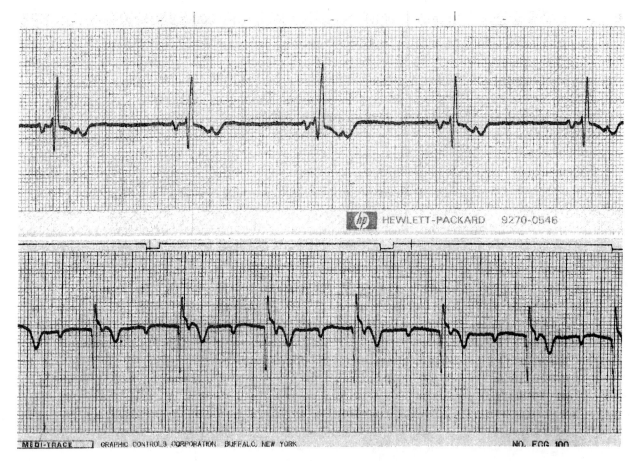

FIGURE 13.2

CASE NUMBER TWO:

The two strips you see in Figure 13.2 are both lead MCL$_1$ and come from separate patients. They are usually presented together in the workshop because these are two arrhythmias that tend to confuse people. Since we like to confuse people in our workshops, we always present them together. They both have instances of 2:1 conduction, but they each occur due to different etiologies. What do you think?

The top strip is a patient whose QRS complex rate is slow. There are two P waves for each QRS complex (one is buried in each T wave). This EKG is representative of one of the most common "causes of pauses," to use a Marriott term. And that is a nonconducted, premature, atrial complex. This patient has premature atrial bigeminy that is nonconducted, creating the slow QRS rate. Each early, nonconducted PAC has delayed the firing of the next P wave, such that it causes a rather slow rhythm. The ultimate management of this patient will involve controlling the atrial activity. However, in the prehospital setting, most EMS organizations do not carry the pharmacologic tools necessary to do that. Consequently, this patient would most likely be treated with atropine.

The bottom strip also has two P waves for each QRS complex, a 2:1 conduction ratio. Is this 2:1 type I or type II? To determine that, we need to analyze the conducted complexes. We find that there is a long PR interval and a narrow QRS complex. So this is a 2:1 type I, in the AV node proper, and is probably benign.

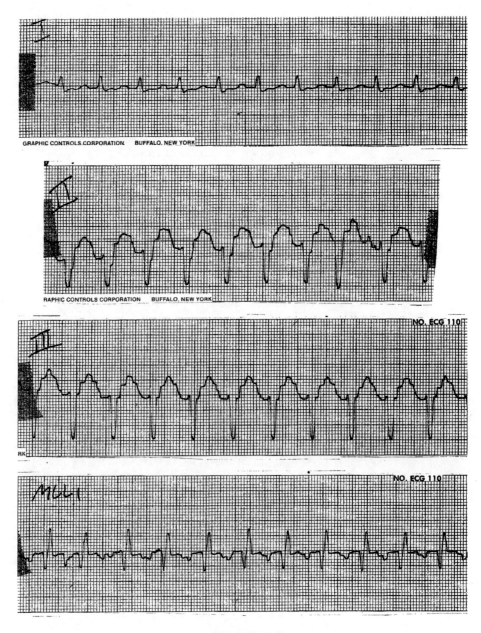

FIGURE 13.3

CASE NUMBER THREE:

Figure 13.3 is the EKG of a 73-year-old male who was awakened from a sound sleep by chest pain and moderate shortness of breath. He is awake, alert, well oriented, and in moderate distress. He describes his pain as "pressure...squeezing-type pain" without radiation. His breath sounds are bilaterally equal with some mild rales in the bases. He has a history of cigarette smoking and hypertension, along with one previous (10-day) hospitalization for a myocardial infarction. He is currently taking nitroglycerin as needed for management of his occasional chest pain and antihypertensive medication.

This patient is in a sinus tachycardia. He has wide QRS complexes. Looking in MCL$_1$, finding the J point, and drawing a line back into the complex reveals an upright triangle. So his wide complexes are due to a right bundle branch block. His axis is a pathologic left axis deviation. So he has a right bundle branch block and a left anterior hemiblock. There is also some S-T segment elevation in leads II and III, indicating the possibility of an evolving inferior wall myocardial infarction. With his precursors to complete heart block, this patient may be a candidate for a pacemaker. He may also be a candidate for thrombolytic therapy for his myocardial infarction.

CASE NUMBER FOUR:

Figure 13.4 is one of my favorite EKGs of all times. A student brought this to me during a class several years ago. Normally, we include it as the last EKG during the posttest of the workshop. This strip is normally accompanied by the message that "if you can diagnose this electrocardiogram, I'll buy you lunch."

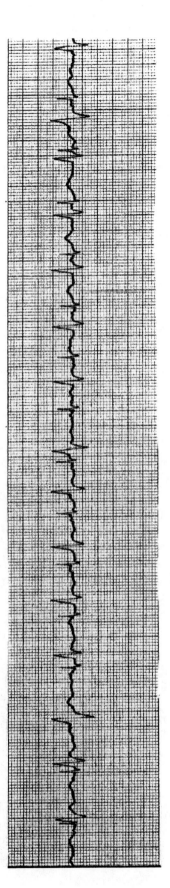

FIGURE 13.4

This is a lead II electrocardiogram. This patient had a history of severe heart failure. But the heart that they were going to transplant into this patient was inadequate to support his entire system. So they left his original heart in place and transplanted an additional heart in, piggyback style. So this patient actually has two hearts in his chest. Usually, when I reveal this information, I get lots of boo and hisses from the audience.

CASE NUMBER FIVE:

A film crew from one of the Denver news stations was riding along on our ambulance for the evening. They had been doing a week-long profile of the Denver Paramedic Division, and they had film footage on everything that they had wanted except for coverage of a shooting or stabbing! So our supervisor met us at the beginning of the shift and told us that we were going to be positioned in the downtown area and were going to respond to all the shootings and stabbings in the city that evening. We would be considered "out of service" for "routine" calls that shift. As you can imagine, we thought this sounded like a pretty fun way to spend the evening. But soon after we loaded the film crew in back, the system got very busy. So we were asked to respond to a nonemergency call just a few blocks away from where we were prowling, on "a sick case."

We arrived to find a 70-year-old male sitting on his bed with a chief complaint of "I've been drinking water all day." That was his only complaint. And, despite all kinds of questioning, the only other information we were able to obtain was that he had been to Denver General's emergency department five times that week for the same complaint, "and they haven't done anything for me yet!" Our secondary survey found the patient to be alert and able to answer questions quite rationally. His skin was warm and dry, with only slightly pale color. His blood pressure was 140/70, his respiratory rate was 24, and he had a slightly irregular pulse rate of 90. He had an oxygen tank in the house, but he wasn't wearing his nasal cannula ("I save it for when I really need it"). He had a large collection of COPD-type medications. And he had a cocked and loaded 38 caliber revolver under the pillow of his bed (a little bit of street survival assessment is important even when you're doing "EKG stuff"). We ran an electrocardiogram and obtained the leads I, II, III, and MCL_1 that you see in Figure 13.5.

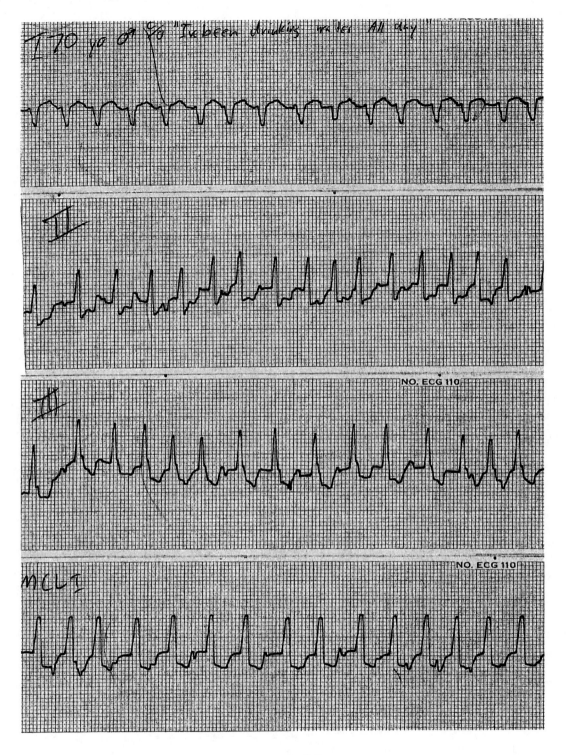

FIGURE 13.5

This electrocardiogram is a tachycardia with a right axis deviation. The QRS complexes are 0.10 seconds wide, so they aren't quite wide enough for a bundle branch block. With upright complexes in MCL_1 and a right axis deviation, there is a good chance this patient has right ventricular hypertrophy. If you look at the rhythm, it is irregularly irregular. Some people see this strip and insist they see P waves between the QRS complexes, but admit that they have different shapes. So there's probably two reasonable diagnoses for this rhythm. One would be atrial fibrillation with a rapid ventricular response. The other one, which is very common in severe COPD, would be multifocal atrial tachycardia.

When we got this patient to the hospital, they drew a blood sample and found him to have a toxic level of theophylline. Once that was discovered, the emergency department staff began asking him more specific questions.

This gentleman had recently been feeling more and more short of breath. And each time he felt short of breath, he took one of his Theodur tablets (using his oxygen only occasionally). As it turns out, there were times when he was taking a tablet approximately every 30 or 40 minutes! Since xanthine (theophylline) derivatives induce diuresis, this man was dehydrated from frequent urination and "drinking water all day." Unfortunately, each of the five previous times he went to the hospital, both he and the receiving staff had been ineffective at communicating. Thus, he hadn't received an adequate evaluation, and they hadn't discovered how truly sick he was.

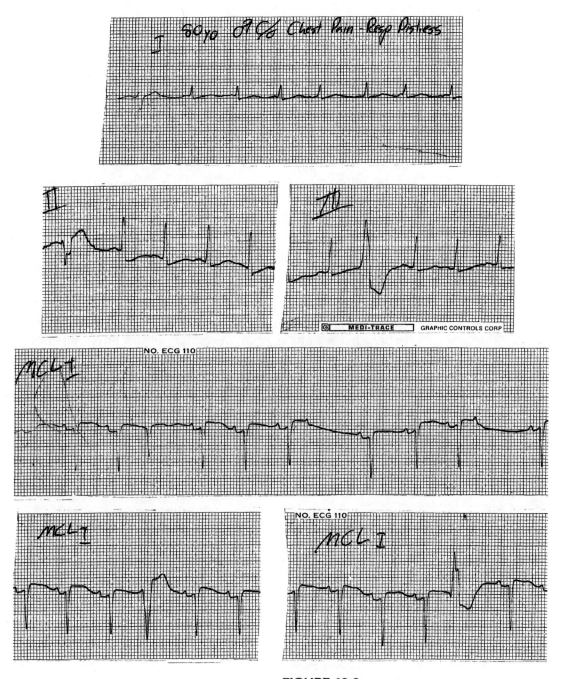

FIGURE 13.6

CASE NUMBER SIX:

An 80-year-old male called 911 complaining of chest pain and respiratory distress. He had a history of angina controlled with occasional nitroglycerin. He had been a one pack a day smoker for over 40 years. We found him to be alert and well oriented, his skin was warm and dry with good color, and he had coarse breath sounds bilaterally. His vital signs were well within normal limits. Figure 13.6 is his EKG; leads I, II, and III, with three sections of MCL_1.

This patient's EKG is a sinus tachycardia with lots of ectopic beats. Let's do an inventory of the various ectopy present: In the first strip of MCL$_1$, the fourth QRS complex is an early, narrow complex without any preceding atrial activity. It's probably a premature junctional contraction. After the seventh and tenth QRS complexes in that strip, there are two incidents of early P waves without QRS complexes—two nonconducted PACs (the most common cause of a pause). In the lower-left MCL$_1$ strip there is a negative, wide QRS complex that's early, with no preceding atrial activity—probably a right ventricular PVC. (We know this PVC is from the right ventricle because the MCL$_1$ electrode is perched just above the right ventricle. Therefore, an impulse that originates there will travel away from the positive MCL$_1$ electrode, producing a negative complex.)

In the lower-right MCL$_1$ strip there is an early complex that is upright with a left rabbit ear taller than the right. It is a left ventricular PVC. (We know this PVC is from the left ventricle because the MCL$_1$ electrode is perched just above the right ventricle, opposite to the left ventricle. Therefore, an impulse that originates in the left ventricle would travel toward the positive MCL$_1$ electrode, producing an upright complex.) This patient has a sinus rhythm, normal axis, with atrial, junctional, and multifocal ventricular ectopy. He should receive large concentrations of oxygen, an IV line, and pain control. Depending on the success of these treatments, local protocols should dictate his management with lidocaine.

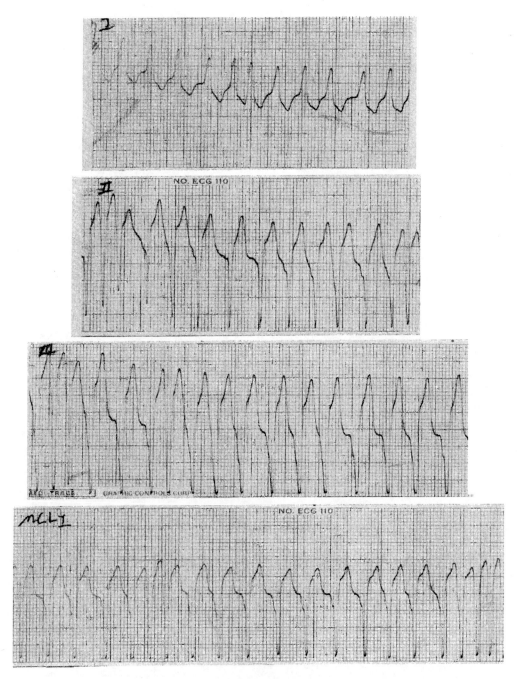

FIGURE 13.7

CASE NUMBER SEVEN:

Figure 13.7 is the EKG of a 35-year-old male whose only complaint is that of feeling "different" today. He then mentions he has a history of WPW and is taking quinidine. He has a blood pressure of 98/60, an irregular pulse of 72, and a respiratory rate of 26, with bilaterally clear and equal breath sounds. He is anxious, but alert and well oriented, and his skin is slightly pale, but warm and dry.

This patient has a very fast, wide rhythm that is irregularly irregular. You've seen this EKG before (in Chapter Nine), but it is one that bears repeating. When you see a wide complex tachycardia that persists in being irregularly irregular, you should be thinking "atrial fibrillation with aberrancy." When the rate of this irregularly irregular wide complex tachycardia exceeds 300 beats per minute at times (as it does at the beginning of lead III and the end of MCL$_1$ in Figure 13.7), you should be thinking WPW. It generally requires supraventricular impulses traveling accessory pathways to accomplish that kind of rate. There are several different methods of treating this particular arrhythmia. We elected to use synchronized cardioversion and were successful in this particular case.

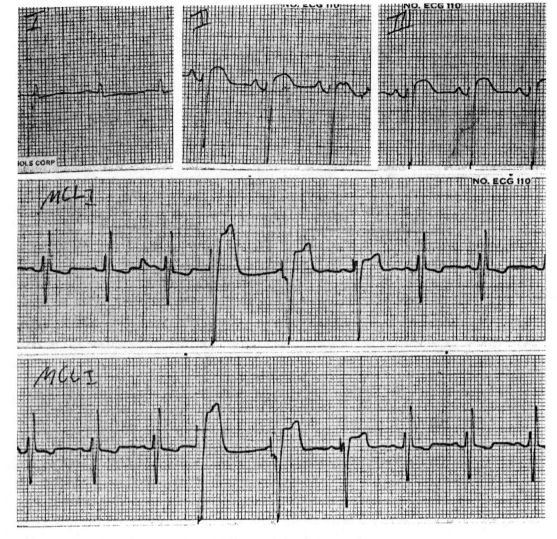

FIGURE 13.8

CASE NUMBER EIGHT:

A 69-year-old male was awakened from a sound sleep by "crushing" chest pain "just like my other heart attack." He feels short of breath and also complains of pain in his left armpit and the left side of his neck. His "heart attack" was three years ago, resulting in a lengthy hospital stay, and he's been on Diazide ever since. He reports taking two Nitrostat prior to calling 911. The nitro gave him a headache and didn't diminish his chest pain at all. In addition to all this, he mentions that his bouts of exertional-onset angina have been fairly frequent for some time, but usually relieved by rest alone.

This patient is alert and well oriented, with pale, cool, moist skin. His lung sounds are bilaterally clear and equal. His blood pressure is 140/84, his pulse 90 and slightly irregular, and his respiratory rate is 20 without obvious signs of distress. Figure 13.8 is his electrocardiogram.

Anyone who is awakened from a sound sleep by chest pain should be considered to be having cardiogenic chest pain, until proven otherwise. This gentleman also reports that the pain is exactly the same as his previous MI—a good clue. Remember that diagnosis and treatment of acute myocardial infarction should be based primarily upon patient *history*. The electrocardiogram may be helpful to "rule in" an infarction, but a "*normal*" EKG cannot "rule out" AMI.

Figure 13.8 is a sinus rhythm with a left axis deviation (a probable left anterior hemiblock) and a right bundle branch block (evidenced by the RSR´ morphology with QRS complex width greater than 0.12 seconds). Each MCL_1 strip has a group of three funny looking beats. The first FLB is early and wide, without preceding atrial activity, and primarily negative in deflection. Thus, the first FLB of each group is probably a right ventricular PVC. The second and third FLBs are each preceded by a little spike—a pacemaker spike. Well, of course he forgot to mention that he had a pacemaker! And how often do we specifically ask about pacemakers before seeing spikes on the EKG (or finding the battery lump of the older models)? Not often. But, there's nothing wrong with that, as long as we notice when a pacemaker problem exists. Does this patient have a pacemaker problem? No, he doesn't.

The compensatory pause that followed the PVC was long enough for the patient's demand right ventricular pacemaker to sense the need to fire. It fired an impulse just as the patient's sinus node resumed. Thus, the combination of impulses—one from the artificial pacemaker and one from the sinus node—blended together to create a fusion beat. Recall that a fusion beat is halfway between a PVC and a normal beat. This is FLB number two. Then there was another pause, followed by another combination of artificial and natural pacemaker impulses, producing another fusion beat (FLB number three). The presence of spikes and fusion beats testifies to the patient's pacemaker appropriately sensing, firing, and capturing. There is no pacemaker problem here. But there is occasional ectopy.

Should you consider lidocaine for this patient? He has demonstrated precursors to complete heart block (left anterior hemiblock and right bundle branch block). But he has also demonstrated the presence of the definitive treatment for complete heart block—a properly functioning pacemaker. So, yes, if your protocols called for it and the patient didn't improve with oxygen and pain control, lidocaine could be administered.

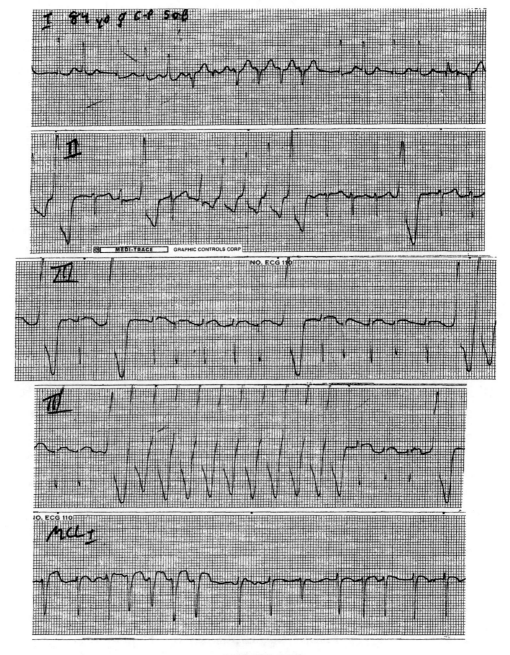

FIGURE 13.9

CASE NUMBER NINE:

The electrocardiogram in Figure 13.9 is one of the more complex EKGs presented in this text. That's why I saved it for the very last.

This EKG is that of an 84-year-old female who had an onset of chest pain and shortness of breath while watching a passionate soap opera. She is awake and alert. Her pulse is 110 and irregular, her blood pressure is 110/60, and her respiratory rate is 28. Her skin is slightly cool, slightly moist, and slightly pale. She has a history of a couple previous strokes and is on Coumadin to manage her clotting problems.

On evaluation, her electrocardiogram shows two different rhythms. The underlying rhythm is atrial fibrillation with a rapid ventricular response. Her underlying beats show a pathologic left axis deviation with a little q wave in lead I and a little r wave in lead III, indicating an anterior hemiblock. The other runs of beats in her EKG have a right axis deviation, so that does not help a lot. But they are wide and quite bizarre and have perfectly regular runs. Their complexes are predominantly negative in MCL_1, so these are right ventricular ectopic beats, with runs of right ventricular tachycardia.

In lead II there is a nice run of V tach that produces fusion as it builds up. Combining with the underlying beats, this run shows progressively more of the ventricles captured by the ectopic ventricular focus.

Treatment for this patient is particularly complex. Because of the atrial fibrillation, lidocaine is problematic, especially when the ventricular response is so rapid. Probably, the best approach is to use something that will address both atrial and ventricular ectopy safely. Procainamide (Pronestyl) will address both atrial and ventricular rates, but (like lidocaine) it has a variable effect upon the A-V node and may speed A-V conduction.[1] Thus, procainamide administration is just as problematic as lidocaine. Beta blocker administration, propranolol (Inderal), may be considered. Propranolol slows A-V conduction and is both an atrial and ventricular antiarrhythmic.[2] The bottom line is this; consult your base physician and follow local protocols.

SUMMARY

It is inevitable that, in the EKG workshops, time runs out before everyone is ready for it to do so. Likewise, each book must end. The world of sophisticated EKG interpretation (for example, using more than lead II!—and everything else in this book) is exciting, especially when your patients benefit. It is always a pleasure to know medical providers who are willing to make an effort to improve patient outcome. Believe me, it's worth it. Happy reading!

REFERENCES

1. *Drug Facts and Comparisons*, J. B. Lippincott Co., St. Louis, MO: 1992; procainamide, pp. 145g–k.
2. *Drug Facts and Comparisons*, J. B. Lippincott Co., St. Louis, MO: 1993; propranolol, pp. 158, 159a–159b.

APPENDIX

Figures to Photocopy, Reduce, and Keep Handy in the Field

Axis (Quick and Easy)

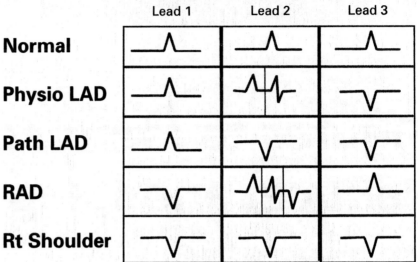

	Lead 1	Lead 2	Lead 3
Normal			
Physio LAD			
Path LAD			
RAD			
Rt Shoulder			

FIGURE 3.9

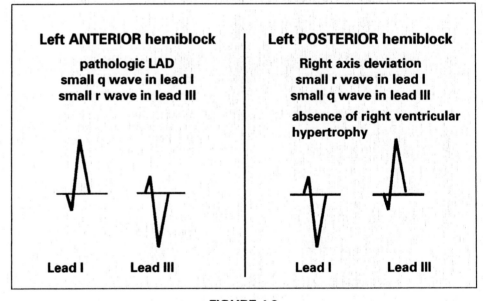

Left ANTERIOR hemiblock

pathologic LAD
small q wave in lead I
small r wave in lead III

Lead I   Lead III

Left POSTERIOR hemiblock

Right axis deviation
small r wave in lead I
small q wave in lead III

absence of right ventricular hypertrophy

Lead I   Lead III

FIGURE 4.3

YES	NO
Absence of an RS Complex (Precordial Leads)	
VT	↓
R-S Interval > 100 ms in 1 Precordial Lead	
VT	↓
A-V DISSOCIATION	
VT	↓
Morphologic Criteria for VT in Vf, V2, V8	
VT	SVT with Aberration

Algorithm for differentiating V tach from SVT with aberration.

Classic Signs of Digitalis Toxicity

1. "If you've got a patient with a bizarre EKG and she's *not* on digitalis, she probably should be. And if you've got a patient with a bizarre EKG and she's *on* digitalis, she is probably on too much of it!"

2. Bidirectional ventricular tachycardia.

Patterns for Recognizing Infarctions

Indicative changes (Q waves, S-T elevation, T wave inversion)

      Anterior MI: leads I, aVL, (V_2, V_3, V_4, V_5

      Lateral MI: leads I, aVL, V_5, V_6

      Inferior MI: leads II, III, aVF

Reciprocal changes (tall and/or broad R waves)

      Posterior MI: leads V_1 and V_2

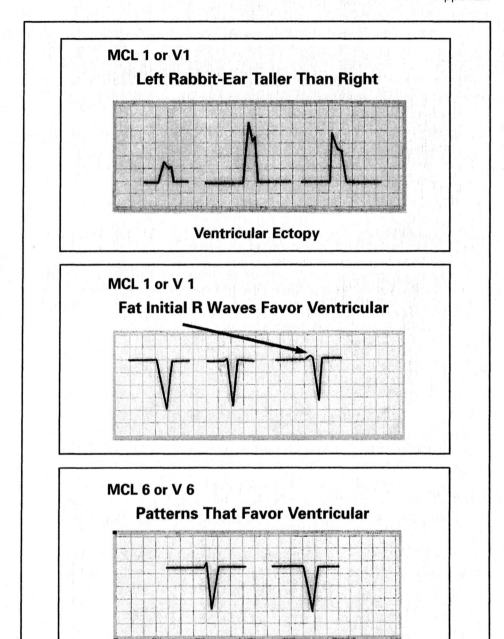

Morphological clues highly suggestive of V tach.

Q-T Interval Norms

Bradycardias may normally have long Q-T intervals. Tachycardias may have short Q-T intervals.

But within normal rates (60 to 110), the Q-T interval should be half the distance of the preceding R-R interval.

If it is longer, suspect hypocalcemia.

Index